Practice Professional Development Planning

Practice Professional Development Planning

A guide for primary care

Peter Wilcock
Chartered Clinical Psychologist
Visiting Fellow in Healthcare Improvement
Institute of Health and Community Studies
Bournemouth University

Charles Campion-Smith
General Practitioner, Cornwall Road Practice, Dorchester
Associate Lecturer in Primary Care Education and Development
Institute of Health and Community Studies
Bournemouth University

and

Sue Elston
Practice Manager, St Alban's Medical Centre, Bournemouth
Educational Facilitator, Centre for General Practice
Institute of Health and Community Studies
Bournemouth University

Foreword by

Professor Sir Kenneth Calman
Vice Chancellor and Warden, University of Durham
Former Chief Medical Officer, England

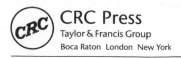

CRC Press
Taylor & Francis Group
Boca Raton London New York

CRC Press is an imprint of the
Taylor & Francis Group, an **informa** business

Radcliffe Medical Press Ltd
18 Marcham Road
Abingdon
Oxon OX14 1AA
United Kingdom

www.radcliffe-oxford.com
The Radcliffe Medical Press electronic catalogue and online ordering facility.
Direct sales to anywhere in the world.

British Library Cataloguing in Publication Data

A catalogue record for this book is available from the British Library.

ISBN 978 1 85775 805 4

Typeset by Advance Typesetting Ltd, Oxfordshire

Contents

Foreword   7

Preface   9

About the authors   11

Acknowledgements   13

Introduction to the guide   **15**

What does the guide contain?   15
How should the guide be used?   17
The PPDP as a learning process   18
Preparing to use the guide   18

Part One: Some underlying thoughts   **19**

What is practice professional development   19
   planning (PPDP)?
Background and context to PPDPs   20
Our approach to PPDP   21
How will this guide help you and your team?   23
The PPDP   24
Personal development plans (PDPs) and PPDPs   25
Summary   26

Part Two: Introduction to the PPDP framework   **27**
and the portfolio

Introduction   27
The PPDP framework   27
Holding interprofessional meetings within the practice   30
The PPDP portfolio   31
Stages of the PPDP process   31
Reviewing progress during the year   33

**Part Three: The stages of the PPDP process
and the portfolio**   **35**

Introduction   35
Stage 1: Discovering priority needs   36
Stage 2: Choosing areas for improvement   39
Stage 3: Agreeing specific actions for improvement   42
Stage 4: Agreeing learning and development needed   46
    to achieve improvements
Stage 5: Planning for reviewing progress of the   50
    PPDP during the year
Stage 6: Planning next year's PPDP   53

Part Four: Some useful tips and resources   **55**

A guide to reflecting on the PPDP process   55
A brief introduction to the principles and methods   57
    of CQI
One practice's story of team learning with PPDP   65
Personal development plans (PDPs)   76
Facilitating PPDP meetings: learning from   84
    our experience
SWOT analysis   88
Significant event analysis (SEA): a summary   91

References   97
Index   101

Foreword

Professions have a number of characteristics in common, amongst which two are of particular interest to the notion of practice development plans. The first is a special relationship with those whom they serve – patients, in the case of health professionals. The second is the concept of self regulation and the ability to assure the public that the doctor, nurse, physiotherapist etc. are fit to practise. Both of these characteristics are captured in the concept of practice development plans. These plans are first of all directed at improving the quality of care to patients and the health of the public. Second, they are about ensuring that all professionals are up to date and aware of new developments in practice.

Over the years, self regulation has been practised in many different ways. Individual professional groups have meetings, case conferences, audit, clinical reviews, and many other activities, all of which were designed to question existing practice and to improve it. With the increasing development of team-based practice it was an obvious step to use the team as the focus for learning and improving patient care. Hence the development of the practice-based planning process, a potentially very powerful way of ensuring change and improvement.

Such a process is not new and is already happening in many places. However, the more systematic approach adopted in this guide allows its wider application, and for those not already involved, it provides a very useful way to start the process.

The guide begins by defining the problems or tasks to be undertaken. Such methods are particularly useful in that they identify real issues which are relevant to a wide group of health professionals and to which everyone can contribute. The learning is therefore both *about* the problem itself, but also *from* each other, as the different professional expertise is brought to bear on a particular problem. It is outcome focused on the needs of patients and the community, and thus on overall improvement in care. If several topics are chosen each year and acted upon, then over a period of several years there will be a significant improvement in patient care across the practice. Indeed, the mere fact that such a process exists stimulates a regular review of practice in other areas.

A major constraint put forward is that of time. How can we find the time to do this? Experience shows that such a process may even save time as new methods of working may make the practice more efficient as well as more effective. There is also the concern that such practice-based planning might get in the way of personal development plans. Again, experience suggests that the two are not incompatible and indeed support each other.

Any remaining doubts should be expelled by a look at the examples given in this guide. They bring the whole process to life and show how learning in teams and sharing of experience can add to the quality of care provided. This must be one of the objectives of all professional groups and if, at the same time, it enhances professional roles and is associated with personal development then it is of all-round benefit. This guide shows how it can be done, and how such benefits can be achieved. The objective, after all, is to serve our patients and the community more effectively.

Professor Kenneth Calman
Vice Chancellor and Warden
University of Durham
Former Chief Medical Officer, England
March 2003

Preface

We are very pleased to welcome you to this guide, which has grown out of our work at the Institute of Health and Community Studies, Bournemouth University with general practices, mainly in Dorset, over a period of several years. In the early days our focus was on the use of the principles and methods of continuous quality improvement within primary care and this then broadened more explicitly into the use of these methods by interprofessional teams within practices.[1]

One of the questions that surfaced regularly was how we could move our work from special projects with external funding to mainstream activity that is part of everyday practice, and which involves everybody within the practice. We were aware that unless both of these were achievable the goal of continuous improvement itself could not be achieved.

We were very excited therefore when Sir Kenneth Calman proposed the idea of practice professional development plans (PPDPs) in 1998.[2] Not only were the underlying principles of his idea congruent with the work we had been undertaking but we felt that the methods we had been exploring would lend themselves well to supporting the implementation of PPDPs, as well as giving them a clear 'needs'-based focus. One of our early lessons, quite appropriately, had been that if you want busy staff to devote time to activities it had to be clear that this would be an investment that would provide benefits for patients.

We experimented with the ideas for a while, influenced by Deming's ideas about organisations as systems, and developed an initial framework for preparing PPDPs (*see* Deming WE (1993) *The New Economics*. MIT Press, Cambridge, MA). We were looking for a way to connect patient and community needs, continuous quality improvement methods and adult learning principles. Our goal was to establish a process that would allow individual and practice development plans to be linked to the practice's agreed improvement priorities, which in turn could clearly be traced back to an exploration of the needs of the practice's patients and local community. In addition these days it is crucial to take into account externally-imposed government, strategic health authority (SHA) and primary care trust (PCT) targets.

We were fortunate to obtain funding to test the framework out with a small cohort of practices within Dorset. We learned a lot and the feedback was positive enough to test things out further with a second small group, this time from different parts of the region. The feedback remained positive and the framework helped create PPDPs that produced benefits for practices and those that depended on them. At the same time the framework was introduced more broadly across Dorset where approximately half the practices now use it to guide their practice professional development planning.

One regular request has been to provide structured guidance for those wishing to use the approach. This guide has been prepared in response to such requests. It is neither a cookbook nor a textbook but contains the distillation of our learning from the practices with which we have worked. In many ways it is a celebration of their work and we are very grateful to them for having been prepared to act as test beds for the future.

Peter Wilcock
Charles Campion-Smith
Sue Elston
March 2003

About the authors

Peter Wilcock BSc, Dip Psych, MSc, PGCert (THE), C Psychol, FBPsS, ILTM is a Chartered Clinical Psychologist with over 20 years of clinical and managerial experience in the NHS. Since 1993, he has been a member of the academic staff at the Institute of Health and Community Studies at Bournemouth University, where he is Visiting Fellow in Healthcare Improvement. His special interest is linking the principles and methods of continuous quality improvement with interprofessional learning in practice settings. He is an advisor to the NHS Modernisation Agency on using patient narratives to drive improvement in care.

He publishes regularly in the field of healthcare improvement and interprofessional learning and is a member of the Editorial Board of the *Journal of Interprofessional Care*, being joint Guest Editor of a special edition about continuous quality improvement in May 2000.

Charles Campion-Smith MB ChB, DCH, FRCGP has been a General Practitioner in Dorchester, Dorset for 23 years. He is Associate Lecturer in Primary Care Education and Development at the Institute of Health and Community Studies at Bournemouth University.

He has been involved in education for more than 10 years, initially as GP Tutor and more recently working with interprofessional primary care teams, using a continuous quality improvement approach to help teams design and bring about improvement in the services they offer their patients.

He has published papers on general practitioner education, interprofessional learning and continuous quality improvement in primary care.

Sue Elston MA, MIMgt, FAETC, AMSPAR Dip is a Practice Manager for a five-doctor partnership in Bournemouth and is seconded to the Institute of Health and Community Studies, Bournemouth University, as an Educational Facilitator in primary care. She has been involved in education in general practice for the past 10 years and since completing her MA in Interprofessional Health and Community Care has developed a keen interest in interprofessional education and development.

She presented her MA dissertation at the 4th International Qualitative Research Conference in Canada in 2000 and the work was published in the *Journal of Interprofessional Care*. Over the past two years her work has included facilitating the process of practice professional development planning for around 60 practices across Dorset and the surrounding area.

Acknowledgements

The work on which this guide is based has taken place at the Institute of Health and Community Studies, Bournemouth University, over several years with financial support from Dorset Health Authority, Wessex Deanery and the South West Region NHS Executive.

Sue Elston's work facilitating practices in practice professional development planning (PPDP) was supported by Wessex Deanery and Bournemouth University as the Educational Facilitator Project.

We thank the following for their support:

- Dr David Percy, former Wessex Director of Postgraduate GP Education
- Howard Nattrass, former Head of School, Institute of Health and Community Studies
- Steve Annandale and Sheila McCann, South West Region NHS Executive.

To the practices in Dorset and throughout the south west of England who worked with us, tried out and refined these ideas, special thanks. Thanks also to the Dorset GP Tutor and Associate Advisor Team for their support.

Tom Hopkins gave us much help in translating the work into a readable and accessible format and Natasha Young has provided secretarial help and technical expertise over several years; we thank them both.

We are grateful to our colleagues at the Institute of Health and Community Studies and those from further afield who have questioned and commented on this work and helped us clarify and, we hope, improve how we describe it.

We thank Professor Sir Kenneth Calman for both providing the initial inspiration for this work and for writing the fore-word to the guide.

The chapter 'One practice's story of team learning with PPDP' was first published in the Quality Supplement of the *British Journal of General Practice* (October 2002) and is used here with permission of the editors. The chapter on continuous quality improvement is adapted from Wilcock and Campion-Smith[3] and is used with permission of the editors. The section on sig-nificant event analysis is based on the work of Dr Jonathan Stead and colleagues at Exeter and we thank them for generously sharing this.

Thank you to Alex Hallatt for her wonderful cartoons.

Feedback please!

As educational developers we are keen to learn from your experi-ences of using this guide – both what went well and what needs improving. Please contact us at the address below. Our thanks in advance for doing so.

Peter Wilcock, Charles Campion-Smith and Sue Elston
Institute of Health and Community Studies
Bournemouth University
Royal London House
Christchurch Road
Bournemouth BH1 3LT
E-mail ccampions@aol.com

Introduction to the guide

Welcome to *Practice Professional Development Planning (PPDP): a guide for primary care*. The guide is the outcome of a development project on PPDP, supported by the South West Region NHS Executive, and undertaken during the period 1998–2001 by the authors. It has been designed to help practice staff in planning and undertaking the tasks and activities involved in PPDP. In particular, the guide should prove helpful to those staff with special responsibility for leading and/or facilitating the PPDP process within their work setting.

What does the guide contain?

The guide contains a number of information and learning resources:

- background information and context of PPDP
- information about key elements, structures and processes in PPDP and related concepts
- points between each stage designed to help you reflect about progress and identify activities still to be undertaken, or things that might be better done differently
- a case example of PPDP in action, the Maples Practice, which is a composite based on the experience of the different practices involved in the early work
- references to recommended and suggested further reading listed in Part Four.

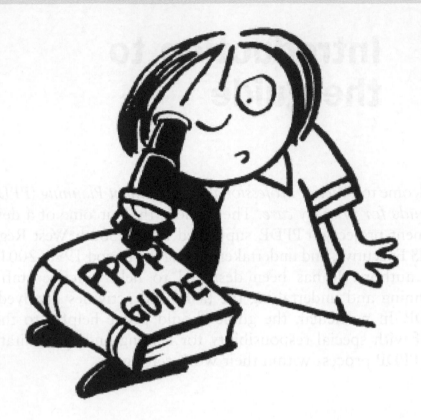

Another feature of this guide is that it is based on key learning principles. By using these as cornerstones for the content and structure, the guide will:

- help you review current work experiences as a starting point for new learning
- assist you in integrating new ideas, concepts and methods with your existing knowledge and skills
- help prepare you for new working situations
- help you develop new skills, or use existing skills in new ways
- help you identify and check your own skill and knowledge development
- contribute to achieving your personal and team learning aims and objectives.

How should the guide be used?

The guide is intended primarily to help team or group-based learning. However, it is highly likely that in busy practices there will be times when it is difficult, if not impossible, for all staff to work together simultaneously on developmental tasks. In this case the guide can provide a useful framework for absent staff to keep abreast of colleagues' learning activities, and a means of support in catching up with recent developments.

However the process we describe is a logical progression. It has been most successful when followed in a stepwise manner, with work to discover and understand the needs of the patients, the local community and the practice as the foundation for the later stages. Our experience has been that it is worthwhile resisting the urge to rush to answers and action. Spending time reflecting on what you know about the current situation before agreeing team aims is essential.

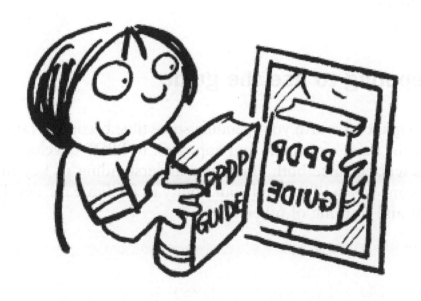

The PPDP as a learning process

We see the PPDP process as the practice team learning together and believe that reflecting on the experience of undertaking it is a vital part of its development within the practice. It is important that the team proceeds with its PPDP on the basis of common understanding of key issues. Therefore if your team is new to PPDP we suggest you all briefly review your understanding of the information and concepts presented.

It is also well worthwhile allocating 15 minutes at the end of each workshop to reflect back on its content and process. This will be most beneficial if it is both a team and individual process and will help to identify any gaps in current understanding and enable the team to proceed with confidence. Some key questions to help are included in Part Four of the guide. It is worth noting that records of such reflections may well make a useful contribution to the PPDP and individual staff learning portfolios.

Preparing to use the guide

We suggest it's worth you spending some time becoming familiar with the guide's contents and approach to PPDP development. This will enhance both your own understanding of key ideas and concepts in PPDP, and your ability to facilitate the development and learning of others.

PART ONE:

Some underlying thoughts

What is practice professional development planning (PPDP)?

For the purposes of this guide, the following definition of PPDP is used:[2]

> A Practice Professional Development Plan describes the developments planned, and the specific educational actions for individuals, groups and the whole team to enable the Practice to improve care, and which is reviewed annually.

Although PPDPs may sound terrifying they only describe activities that are already happening in the majority of practices. The PPDP simply brings the activities together in a systemic way and, by linking them to meeting the needs of individuals and communities, enables a more coherent overview to emerge.

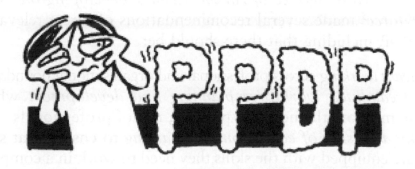

Background and context to PPDPs

PPDPs were first proposed by Sir Kenneth Calman (then Chief Medical Officer) in 1998. According to the paper *A Review of Continuing Professional Development in General Practice*,[2] they would:

- develop the concept of the 'whole practice' as a human resource for healthcare
- be professionally led at all levels, and
- be monitored through peer review.

The essence of the plan was to identify individual and practice learning needs and develop a strategy to meet them. Planning was to be annual for both the individual and the practice, and was to respond to the findings of clinical audit, local needs and objectives, and national priorities.

However, recently completed work had highlighted how traditional GP postgraduate medical education was seldom selected to meet a particular patient or practice need and only changed clinical practice infrequently.[4] Moreover, the requirement to undertake PPDP is but one of a range of current or anticipated demands on general practice and primary care staff time. Clinical governance is already a feature of everyday healthcare, and re-accreditation and revalidation of GPs is on the horizon.

More recently the Department of Health consultation document *A Health Service of All the Talents: developing the NHS workforce*[5] made several recommendations of direct relevance to PPDP, including that there should be:

- *team working* across professional and organisational boundaries
- *streamlined workforce planning and development* which stems from the needs of patients, not of professionals
- *modernising of education and training* to ensure that staff are equipped with the skills they need to work in a complex, changing NHS.

Whilst these requirements present real opportunities to re-examine policy and practice, they also generate additional work for already busy teams. Therefore, there is an imperative to use time for learning effectively in order to satisfy the requirements of governance, educational accreditation and preparation for revalidation. It is in this context that the guide seeks to support and guide staff through PPDP.

Our approach to PPDP

As those responsible for leading the change process within the project, we found ourselves moving from a traditional teaching and telling role to a facilitating one, offering strategies and 'tools' to help practice teams make the most effective use of the wealth of expertise which they already possessed. Some of these tools are listed in Part Four.

We also found that a patient-focused approach encourages teams to work interprofessionally. When they do so their depth of knowledge and understanding of patients and systems of care is striking. The contribution of all team members is valuable within this approach, and we have found real team development and improved relationships to be a consistent outcome of this way of working.[6]

The lessons which we learned from our work with teams during the PPDP project have been reviewed and distilled into the ideas, concepts, principles and practice recommendations that you will find in this guide.

Linking with the practice's decision-making processes

The aim is not to create yet another time-consuming process that adds burden. Professional development planning must help practices to do better what they already have to do and to link this directly to improving patient care.

Within the practice

As has already been said, being rigorous about prioritising and not being too ambitious is crucial. It is also important to think how the process set out in Part Three can best link into what else is happening in the practice – to ensure it is not just an 'add-on'. Can some of the existing practice meetings be used instead for the PPDP process? Whilst the involvement and commitment of the practice team is required to achieve results, this doesn't mean everyone has to be involved in all the meetings. Delegating the detailed work to a small group, with arrangements for reporting back and consulting, is essential. Finally, make sure that this is the *one* process for developing professional develop-ment plans in the practice, and that it replaces existing processes.

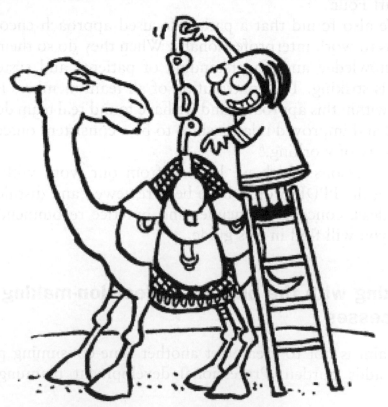

Within the primary care trust (PCT)

The PCT will have, or will be developing, systems for approving and collating professional development plans. These will be influenced increasingly by national policies and practices such as professional re-accreditation. The approach to PPDPs set out in Part Three must link into PCT and national planning processes. It should enable all parties to achieve their objectives of the process and to do so within the timescales laid down each year. It follows that there will be no one way of doing it. Formats for PPDPs and timetables for their production will vary across the country. What is important is that increasingly PPDPs, whatever their precise format, will be based upon a careful team consideration of how better to meet the needs of patients and the local community.

How will this guide help you and your team?

We believe that it is important that the whole primary health-care team (PHCT), both clinical and administrative, is involved with the process of drafting the plan. We have found it is only when the whole team comes together that the full extent of the knowledge and understanding about the activities of a practice becomes apparent.

In what follows here we describe the process that allows a practice to select important areas for development, and to identify the education and training activities and resources required for the whole team and/or individuals.

Freeing up time and resources to dedicate to your PPDP can be difficult. In the pilot stage of our work, teams met on several occasions tackling just one stage of the PPDP process at a time. Feedback suggested that this created problems in attendance

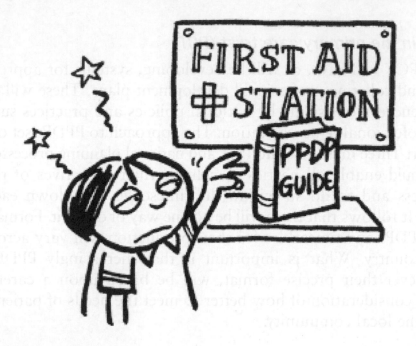

for some members due to work pressures and led to poor continuity. Over time and learning from our experiences we were able to condense the work into two workshops of approximately two and a half to three hours, covering Stages 1–7 of the framework in the first and Stages 8–11 in the second workshop. As long as work is undertaken between meetings to provide the information necessary for the questions being addressed we do not feel that the quality of the work is compromised in any way. Practice teams have found this more realistic and manageable in terms of their time and other work pressures. However the process is flexible enough to allow teams to work at their own pace and to meet as many times as they feel necessary.

The PPDP

The really important part of this approach to PPDPs is the work the team engage in as they progress through the different stages, including the actions they take to bring about improvement. It has been shown time and again that this is usually a major learning experience, and one that frequently transforms team relationships.

Even though this is the most important aspect of the approach, practices will have to produce one or several documents that set out their proposals for professional development. Some primary care trusts (PCTs) will prescribe their format. Others will be content to receive the portfolio of evidence produced as a result of following the stages in Part Three. It is likely that the majority of PCTs will not wish to receive large documents and will opt for a summary of proposals from each practice.

Personal development plans (PDPs) and PPDPs

One of the most frequently asked questions has been about where PDPs fit in with PPDPs in this approach. The simple answer is that they are an integral part.

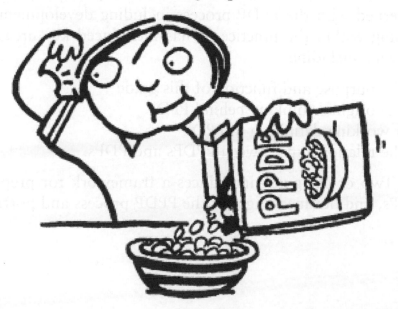

The aim is that an individual's professional development should increasingly be directly related to what they, and other members of the multiprofessional team, have concluded is needed to bring about the improvements in patient care that they have identified as most important. This is what the process set out in Part Three of this guide is designed to achieve.

However, a sense of realism is important here. We recognise that practices can only work on very few areas for improvement in any one year. An individual's learning needs will arise both from the PPDP and from his or her personal practice interests and career aspirations. Similarly learning undertaken as part of the PPDP may well be recorded in an individual's portfolio in preparation for appraisal and revalidation. A framework for PDPs that is congruent with the thinking underpinning this guide is included in Part Four.

Summary

Part One of this guide has covered a number of important issues concerned with the PPDP process including development and learning within the practice. It has introduced key areas and concepts, including:

- the purpose and function of this guide
- the original thinking behind PPDP
- a working definition of PPDP
- the relationship between PPDPs and PDPs.

Part Two of the guide introduces a framework for preparing PPDPs, and outlines stages of the PPDP process and portfolio.

PART TWO:

Introduction to the PPDP framework and the portfolio

Introduction

This part of the guide has five elements:

1   a description of the PPDP framework developed by the authors as the basis for work with practice staff groups and teams
2   a brief overview of important points to consider when holding interprofessional meetings within the practice
3   an introduction to the PPDP portfolio, which is a suggested way of building up the record of your work
4   an introduction to stages of the PPDP process
5   reviewing progress during the year.

The PPDP framework

At first glance the framework may look quite complex, but in reality it simply links a number of activities and processes which are probably already happening in most practices. Advice about working through each stage of the framework is included in Part Three. There are three main elements, explained in the sections immediately below.

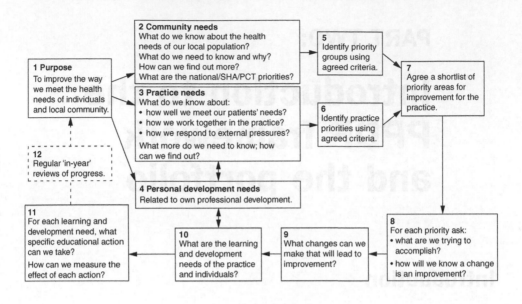

1 Purpose
To improve the way we meet the health needs of individuals and local community.

2 Community needs
What do we know about the health needs of our local population?
What do we need to know and why?
How can we find out more?
What are the national/SHA/PCT priorities?

3 Practice needs
What do we know about:
• how well we meet our patients' needs?
• how we work together in the practice?
• how we respond to external pressures?
What more do we need to know; how can we find out?

4 Personal development needs
Related to own professional development.

5 Identify priority groups using agreed criteria.

6 Identify practice priorities using agreed criteria.

7 Agree a shortlist of priority areas for improvement for the practice.

8 For each priority ask:
• what are we trying to accomplish?
• how will we know a change is an improvement?

9 What changes can we make that will lead to improvement?

10 What are the learning and development needs of the practice and individuals?

11 For each learning and development need, what specific educational action can we take?
How can we measure the effect of each action?

12 Regular 'in-year' reviews of progress.

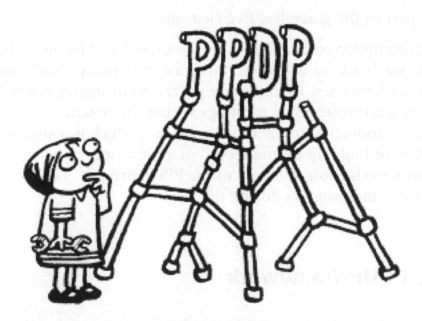

Identifying key developmental priorities for the practice team

These need to be informed by knowledge of the local community, awareness of externally determined and/or driven agendas, requirements (e.g. PCT, health improvement programmes (HImPs), national service frameworks (NSFs) etc.) and inside knowledge of the practice's current working arrangements, and internal/self-assessments (*see* Boxes 1–3 on the framework diagram).

Translating priority areas into planned improvement projects

Continuous quality improvement (CQI)* principles and methods have been used to create an approach to project planning that:

• provides a clear focus for the work to be undertaken
• clarifies who needs to do what and when
• allows the practice team to learn flexibly as they go (*see* Boxes 4–9).

Identifying practice team and individual staff learning needs

The practice's improvement priorities will provide pointers to important team learning needs and in addition new personal and professional development needs will almost certainly arise. A central aim of this approach is to place PDPs firmly in the context of practice improvement priorities. Team members will understand how their PDP fits in with the practice's overall plan to improve the services that it provides. However, there may be parts of some staff members' PDPs which fall outside the PPDP. For example, these aspects of PDPs may relate to professional career plans, or arise from staff appraisal processes, so making them confidential to the individual (*see* Boxes 4 and 10–11).

*An introduction to the CQI approach is included in Part Four, *see* pp 57–64.

Holding interprofessional meetings within the practice

For interprofessional meetings to be useful and productive it is important to pay attention to the process – how people are going to work and learn together. Setting up a meeting of the whole team needs planning. It is really important that people have a clear idea of the aim of the meeting. Telling them the start and finish times and being explicit about what food and refreshments are available allows people to plan.

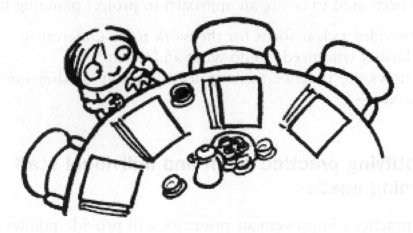

Often the meeting will be more fruitful if people have been asked to consider one or two things in advance. It is important to emphasise the contribution all team members have to make and to acknowledge that for at least some of the participants their prior experience of group working may not have been good. It is very helpful to have a facilitator from outside the practice, particularly for the initial meetings. However one person within the practice will also have to take a leading role in the practicalities of setting the meeting up.

Part of the facilitator's role will be to help the team agree some ground rules about the process of the meetings. The hopes and anxieties of participants, together with previous experience of group work, good and bad, can be used as a starting point for this exercise (*see* Part Four). On pages 84–90 we give some more specific ideas for the facilitation of these meetings.

The PPDP portfolio

By 'portfolio' we just mean a collection of evidence from the learning process the practice team has been going through. It is a suggested way to maintain a record of the information gathered as you move through the steps in the framework and of the decisions the practice team makes about its improvement and learning priorities. In addition it includes evidence which clearly demonstrates what the practice team has learned from drafting its PPDP and from taking the actions required to bring about change and improvement. It is not simply a record of actions, activities or experiences which the team has undertaken but an account of how much value each member of the team feels about having the opportunity to contribute to the direction of the practice. Team members in some practices have valued this aspect of producing the PPDP above all else and have experienced a real improvement in their working relationships. This evidence is certainly worthy of inclusion in the final PPDP document as well as in staff's own personal portfolios.

We have found that a useful format for the portfolio is a loose-leaf ring binder. In it dividers can be used to create sections for each key stage of the PPDP process as shown below.

Stages of the PPDP process

The steps of the PPDP process can usefully be divided into a number of stages which build on each other and which each have a different part to play as they strengthen the practice's ability to improve the way it meets the needs of its patients and local community.

Stage 1 Discovering priority needs (*see* Boxes 1–4 on the framework diagram).

Stage 2 Choosing areas for improvement (*see* Boxes 5–7).

Stage 3 Agreeing specific actions for improvement (*see* Boxes 8–9).

Stage 4 Agreeing learning and development needed to achieve improvement (*see* Boxes 10–11).

Stage 5 Planning for reviewing progress of the PPDP during the year (*see* Box 12).

Stage 6 Planning next year's PPDP.

You will see from the above list that the earlier sections of your portfolio will contain details about how you discovered the needs of your practice. It would also be appropriate to include brief accounts of your PPDP meetings. Later sections will include accounts of how you negotiated and chose areas for action and which team members were involved in these discussions. These sections describe the specific educational and learning activities undertaken by the whole team or by individuals. Some of this material may also be copied and held in individuals' PDPs.

Over time you will find it helpful to gather evidence to show what benefits for patients and/or staff have resulted from the planned changes.

By following the process explained below, your portfolio will establish a body of evidence of your working step by step through the framework. For example, in the section titled 'Discovering priority needs' your evidence could be notes of your first PPDP meeting, listing those present, and a record of what took place. It may also include information about the needs of your local community, externally-determined priorities and the outcome of a SWOT analysis or other evidence identifying the 'current state' with regard to your own internal practice needs.

Reviewing progress during the year

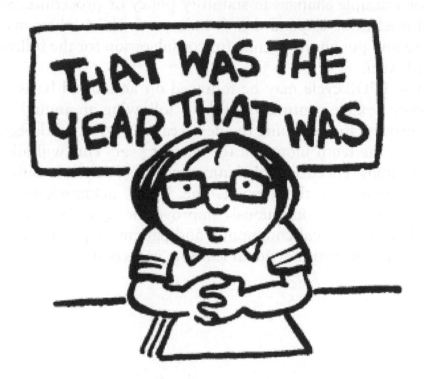

The portfolio approach allows the PPDP and related personal plans to be updated flexibly during the year as circumstances change. It is important that regular reviews of progress are made in order to allow this to happen and opportunities should be planned in at the beginning of each PPDP cycle. It is also often only when a team stops and reflects that they realise just how much they have achieved.

Reviews are also a chance to check that all members of the team are clear about what the purpose of the PPDP is. It is important that while working on a specific topic, team members remember the high level aim of improving the service to the patients and local community. Reconnecting with this and seeing that the specific improvement being worked on is indeed consistent with the high level aim can be encouraging and energising.

These review meetings can also be used to maintain a watching brief on local community needs and external driving forces – for example changes in statutory policy or procedure. Some will need to be responded to 'within year' whilst others may be noted and put on the agenda for consideration for the following PPDP year.

The PPDP cycle may be followed on an annual basis or in a more flexible continuous cycle. If following an annual cycle, the process for designing the next year's PPDP should begin at around the tenth month of the current year. This will allow a continuous reflection and planning process to evolve, with each year building on the previous one. It also acknowledges that for practices to continuously improve the way they meet the needs of their local community and patients a process of continuous team and individual learning is needed.

PART THREE:

The stages of the PPDP process and the portfolio

Introduction

Part Three of this guide introduces the stages of the PPDP process, together with ideas, suggestions and practical examples of how to develop a PPDP portfolio. Each stage is illustrated by composite stories directly drawn from experience with practices involved in the early piloting of the guide.

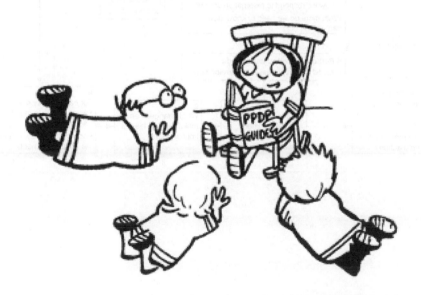

Stage 1: Discovering priority needs

Introduction

This first stage is concerned with the initial aspect of the PPDP process as represented by the first four boxes of the PPDP diagram, as highlighted. It will include how a practice builds knowledge about the needs of its local community and patients as well as highlighting the directives from government, the strategic health authority and the PCT to which it has to respond.

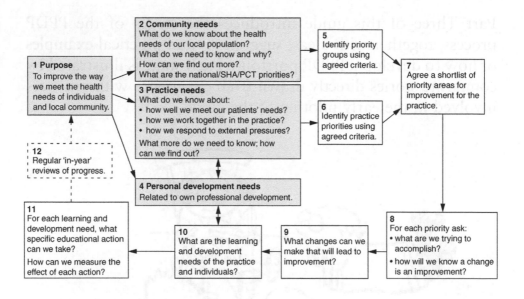

Discovering priority needs

1 Purpose
To improve the way we meet the health needs of individuals, groups and the local community.

2 Community needs
- What do we know about the health needs of the local population?
- What do we need to know and why?
- How can we find out more?
- What are the national/SHA/PCT priorities?

3 Practice needs
What do we know about:
- how well we meet our patients' needs?
- how we work together in the practice?
- how we respond to external pressures?

What more do we need to know; how can we find out?

4 Personal development needs
Related to own professional development.

Purpose

This box simply states the practice's underlying purpose. It reflects the fact that both practice and professional development should be explicitly built on the bedrock of meeting needs, and continuously improve the quality of care for patients.

This PPDP framework has been drawn up to reflect a continuous systemic link between this underlying purpose and the outcomes of individual and team learning plans, thereby linking learning with improving care for patients.

Community needs

You may discover that not all members of the primary healthcare team understand what 'community needs' means and you may have to explain. Check the group's awareness of the following and identify any gaps in knowledge or shortfall in provision:
- local demographics and epidemiology of the practice population
- national priorities i.e. government directives such as 'Our Healthier Nation', national service frameworks
- PCT and Annual Accountability Agreement.

Practice needs

Check the group's knowledge about the practice and the population it serves by looking at:
- specific features of the practice and its population, e.g. access and accessibility
- practice performance indicators such as cervical cytology uptake and adequacy rates, immunisation uptake, prescribing data
- results of self assessment methods such as SWOT analyses, outcome reports and staff views on outcomes of significant event meetings and complaints (see Part 4)
- results of audits or surveys and key findings
- patient and users' views.

Personal development needs

Relevant sections of staff and partner appraisal may identify/clarify areas for improvement in various aspects of practice work.

The Maples Practice story

1 Purpose	2 Community needs	3 Practice needs	4 Personal development needs
To improve the way that we meet the health needs of individuals, groups and the local community.	What do we know about the health needs of the local population? What do we need to know and why? How can we find out more? What are the national/SHA/PCT priorities?	What do we know about: • how well we meet our patients' needs? • how we work together in the practice? • how well we respond to external pressures? What more do we need to know; how can we find out?	Related to own professional development.

Evidence for the portfolio

The Maples Medical Centre serves 10 000 patients and has a primary healthcare team consisting of five doctors, two practice nurses, five community nurses, a health visitor, and 14 management and administrative staff. We used to hold PHCT meetings but these were abandoned due to lack of agenda items and poor attendance. The practice manager has suggested we reinstate the PHCT meetings to work on our PPDP. She believes the PPDP process offers an opportunity for the PHCT to contribute to the future direction of the practice, especially in meeting the needs of our practice population.	A health needs assessment of our practice population had been carried out some years ago and our demography had not changed. However, we were aware that not everyone in the PHCT was familiar with the PCT's priorities and NSFs. A priority for our first PPDP meeting was to present an overview of our local strategic health plan, match this to our practice population, and then identify any gaps in our service provision.	To establish the needs for improvement in the practice we carried out a SWOT analysis. Each member of the PHCT participated and all submissions were sent to the external facilitator for co-ordination. The result was as follows: **Strengths** • Good range of patient services • Good range of skills in PHCT • Meet all targets • Well-organised practice **Opportunities** • To improve the use of IT • To improve patient access • To become a paperless practice **Weaknesses/challenges** • Under-utilisation of computer • Communication could be better • Lack of appointments **Threats** • Time • Money The data not used in the final SWOT was given to the practice manager to follow up. These were mainly management issues to be dealt with outside the PPDP meeting.

Stage 2: Choosing areas for improvement

Introduction

This stage introduces the next three elements of the PPDP process as highlighted in the framework diagram. It often involves a process of negotiation and choice. There are many demands on practices but it is essential that the team is realistic in what it chooses to take on. Issues of high importance or great impact on the life of the practice are likely to command wide support from team members and success with these can help them gain confidence in the process. Once again a real life story from the Maples Practice illustrates how other staff teams have approached these key tasks.

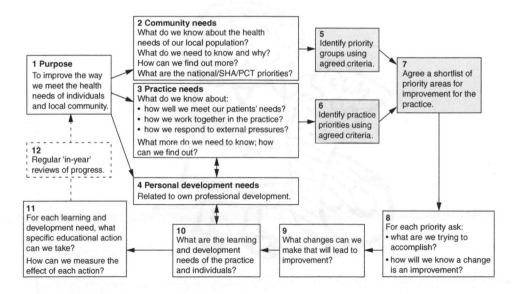

Choosing areas for improvement

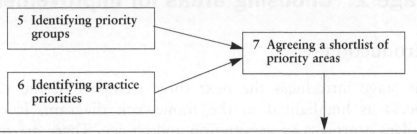

5 Identifying priority groups	
6 Identifying practice priorities	7 Agreeing a shortlist of priority areas

The 'what and why' of identifying priorities and priority areas

• Make sure everyone is aware of the 'external' agenda such as the PCT's priorities and NSFs (see Box 5).
• If the team has carried out individual SWOT analyses, these should be co-ordinated and a compilation of issues identified as requiring attention should be included in the list (see Box 6).
• Do not forget to include the 'must-do's, or the 'it-would-be-foolish-not-to-do's such as addressing health and safety issues or performance targets/indicators. This is where it is important to spend some time reaching agreement on two or three priority areas for improvement to be worked on over the coming year.
• Remember one small change that brings about improvement is worth more than half a dozen good intentions (see Box 7).

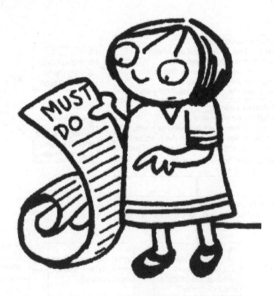

• Finally check your list to make sure that the topics will bring clear benefits to patients and to staff. This requires a balance of priorities between being patient focused and practice focused (see Box 7).

The Maples Practice story

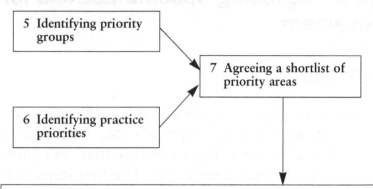

5 Identifying priority groups

6 Identifying practice priorities

7 Agreeing a shortlist of priority areas

Evidence for the portfolio

Representatives from each discipline, nominated by their peers, were invited to a two-hour workshop to discuss and agree priorities for improvement over the next 12 months. A summary of the PCT's priorities, NSFs and the National Primary Care Collaborative (community needs, see Box 5), together with the outcome of the SWOT analysis (practice needs, see Box 6), was presented to the team. Emerging from this data was a long list of potential areas for improvement. Armed with this information and with the help of a facilitator, the team split into two smaller groups to choose three areas we considered to be a priority for the practice and its population.

- To improve and increase the use of IT (in particular data input for chronic disease management). Chosen because we were aware data were being input in a variety of ways rendering audit and search results unreliable. We also had a problem storing increasing amounts of paper and had just had a system upgrade. Our aim would be for 100% of computerised patient records to be complete, accurate and up to date.
- To improve patient access. Chosen because we were already actively participating in the National Primary Care Collaborative and 'access' had been identified as a priority for improvement by the PCT. Our aim would be to offer patients a routine appointment with GP or nurse within 48 hours of request. (Urgent appointment requests were already met on the day.)
- To address the NSF for mental health. Chosen because we were experiencing an increasing number of patients with acute episodes of mental illness requiring medication and who did not come under the care of the community mental health team. These patients required frequent monitoring and support, and the counselling service we provided, with a waiting time of 15 weeks, was inadequate. Our aim would be to provide practice-based support for patients experiencing an acute episode of mental illness.

Stage 3: Agreeing specific actions for improvement

Introduction

This is the stage where the ideas for improvement are translated into action. The CQI approach (*see* Part Four) ensures that there is a clear aim and measures that will show if the action is having the hoped for effect. The first steps to bringing about improvement are planned, tested out and evaluated (*see* Boxes 8 and 9).

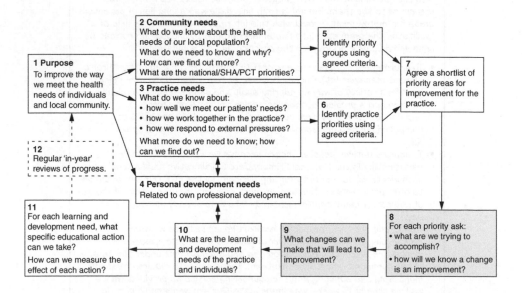

Agreeing specific actions for improvement

8 What are we trying to accomplish? How will we know a change is an improvement?

9 What changes can we make that will lead to an improvement?

For each of your priority high level aims do you need to learn anything more about the current situation, e.g. about patients' needs, the processes by which you currently do things, audit data etc.?

Use whatever you learn from such information to choose small projects that will help you move towards your high level aim for each priority. Agree a specific aim for each project and then choose a few simple measures for each that will provide you with important feedback about the effects of your change.

The 'how' of specific actions for improvement

Agree some simple, practical changes that you can make to accomplish your project aims. It may be helpful to use the plan–do–study–act (PDSA) cycle to guide your activity (see below).

Plan   Set out a plan of action – who will do what and when?

Do   Implement the agreed plans making sure you build in the necessary feedback measures so that you can learn from experience as you go.

Study   Consider the feedback you have collected as well as logs of experience as things have unfolded. What has been learned? What are the implications of this learning for the next steps?

Act   On the basis of what you have learned what will you do next? For example, will you need to change things and carry out another PDSA cycle? Would it be appropriate to extend your trial to more general practice?

As far as possible use rapid, small cycle, changes. Learn fast and build bigger improvements through cumulative, serial changes.

The Maples Practice story

8 What are we trying to accomplish? How will we know a change is an improvement?

9 What changes can we make that will lead to an improvement?

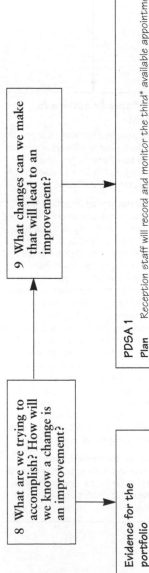

Evidence for the portfolio

Project groups were set up to work on each priority area, and included staff who were not at the PPDP workshop. The aim of the project group for improving access was to accomplish patient appointments within 48 hours', and involved a GP, deputy practice manager and senior receptionist.

They agreed that a change would be an improvement if:

- the number of patients waiting for more than 48 hours decreased
- the new arrangements met patients' needs.

PDSA 1

Plan Reception staff will record and monitor the third* available appointment for each doctor and nurse in order to assess the practice's capacity of doctor and nurse appointments.

Do When a patient requests an appointment the receptionist will record, on a pro-forma, the appointment date the patient requested and the appointment date the patient was given. The reception manager will analyse the data at weekly intervals and record the length of wait for an appointment for each doctor and nurse.

Study Results showed that although the monitoring exercise created additional pressure on reception staff at busy times it was possible to identify peaks in demand, i.e. Mondays and Friday afternoons.

Act To consult about the benefits of introducing one session of nurse triage on Monday mornings.

PDSA 2

Plan To carry out a survey to seek patient views and assess potential use of nurse triage by distributing a simple patient questionnaire to patients attending the surgery and to those receiving repeat prescriptions.

* The third available appointment is a measure of access used by the National Primary Care Collaborative.

Each project group met separately to agree the 'who', 'what' and 'when' and to formulate an action plan. We found that there were usually several cycles of PDSA, e.g. see the box on the right.

Do Reception staff distributed 500 questionnaires and the practice manager monitored and analysed them as they came in.

Study Out of the 430 questionnaires completed, 73% said they would be happy to speak or consult with a nurse in the first instance, 27% of patients said they definitely would not be happy to speak to or consult with a nurse in the first instance.

Act It was decided to proceed with the trial of a weekly session (Monday mornings) of nurse triage.

PDSA 3

Plan To introduce one session per week of nurse triage to be carried out by a newly appointed part-time health visitor who had recently completed the nurse triage course and was keen to maintain her skills. The practice would negotiate with the PCT to allow her to carry out triage for one session per week.

Do Protocols were agreed with doctors. Accommodation, telephone line and computer facilities were organised and the service was advertised in the waiting room and via repeat prescriptions. A patient survey was designed to evaluate patient response to be carried out two months after commencement.

Study The outcome of the patient survey and feedback from the triage nurse, doctors and reception staff indicated that the triage session was alleviating some pressure on appointments at peak times.

Act The Monday morning triage session was confirmed as everyday practice and an additional session was introduced on Friday mornings.

Stage 4: Agreeing learning and development needed to achieve improvements

Introduction

This section is about linking learning with improving care:

* what skills do we need to develop to bring about an improvement in the areas we have identified as a priority
* what do we need to learn, as individuals and as a team, to enable us to deliver the planned improvements?

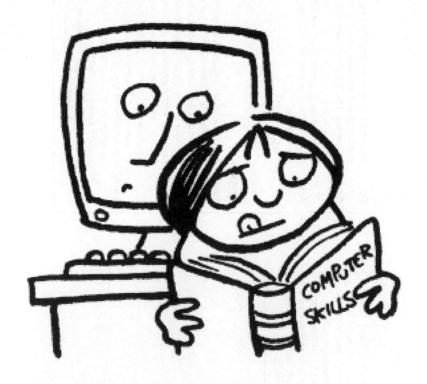

Individual staff may also have personal learning needs in relation to their career development identified separately in the appraisal process.

The Maples Practice story illustrates how other staff teams have approached these key tasks.

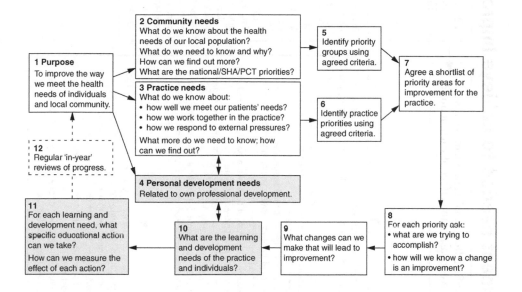

Agreeing learning and development needed to achieve improvements

4 Personal development needs

This refers to individual learning needs and it may be helpful to view these as falling into one or both of the following categories.

- Personal needs – these relate to the outcomes of personal appraisals, revalidation etc. and are confidential. Appraisers need to be aware of PPDP priorities and take them into account during appraisals.
- Organisational needs (see Box 10) – these relate to the PPDP priorities and also core training needs such as annual top ups on health and safety issues, resuscitation, etc. which can be planned ahead. There's no reason why these can't be included in the PPDP and indeed it may prove helpful.

11 What specific educational action can we take? How can we measure the effect of each action?

This refers to specific educational actions taken to meet the improvement. In addition to formally accredited opportunities, you may wish to consider:

- team learning and training events including setting up the process for significant event review and other shared learning events such as the PPDP process
- specific training sessions, for instance resuscitation skills or computer skills – could be away days, clinical attachments or practice-based training sessions
- notes of new systems established to meet a particular need and team learning on how to use these systems
- individual education to attain a specific new skill or knowledge for sharing amongst team members
- personal learning that may come out of an individual's reflection on a particular incident, event, something read or from personal life.

You may also want to note any benefits you feel have resulted from the whole team approach to learning and development such as improved relationships, information sharing, or any change in practice culture. Providing evidence of this is not easy – recording staff comments or incidents, or using relevant sections of staff appraisal may be worthwhile.

A system for sharing with the rest of the team what individuals learn on courses etc. and the implications for the practice.

10 Learning and development needs of the practice and individuals

This will be a list of learning and development needs with respect to the PPDP improvement priorities. It is also necessary to identify the different professionals who will need access to learning opportunities. For the purpose of informing your PCT's education strategy it is also appropriate to list training needs emerging from appraisal.

Not all education and development takes place outside the practice. Indeed, more and more emphasis is being placed on practice-based learning. Recognise the learning that takes place as you work through the PDSA cycles.

The Maples Practice story

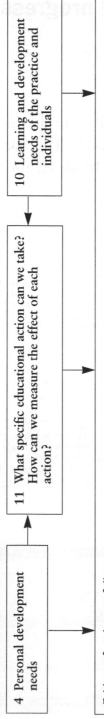

4 Personal development needs

→ 11 What specific educational action can we take? How can we measure the effect of each action?

→ 10 Learning and development needs of the practice and individuals

Evidence for the portfolio

The practice manager was keen to know if the PHCT had found the PPDP process useful. Evaluation of the first workshop indicated that since the PHCT meetings had been abandoned the only time the team got together was at the Christmas party. The opportunity to have time to sit down together to discuss and contribute to the future of the practice was the most positive and valuable outcome of the exercise.

Examples of what needs to be learned

Improve patient access

- The practice nurse requires telephone consultation skills.
- Reception team requires knowledge of telephone consultation and how it fits with their role.
- Educate patients in the use of telephone consultation.

Increase use of computer

- Medical system training for relevant members of the PHCT in use of chronic disease management (CDM) templates, audit, NHSnet training for GPs and use of e-mail for PHCT.

In addition to the training needs emerging from the PPDP the PHCT also has training needs arising from annual appraisal (non-clinical staff) and personal development review (nurses):

- resuscitation skills update
- health and safety update
- risk assessment/risk management update
- desktop publishing
- handling difficult people
- supervisory skills.

The GPs are working on their individual learning plans which will include learning needs associated with the PPDP. For example, a GP, and sessional clinical assistant in A&E, wanted to improve his resuscitation skills, so he put this in his PDP. The PCT in which he works had recently notified practices of their responsibility in providing adequate equipment and skills in practice to deal with patients requiring resuscitation. This is a good example of the link between a doctor's personal development needs and the practice's development needs.

Stage 5: Planning for reviewing progress of the PPDP during the year

Introduction

This stage emphasises the importance in PPDP of undertaking regular reviews of progress within each yearly cycle. The accompanying practice story illustrates an approach to doing so.

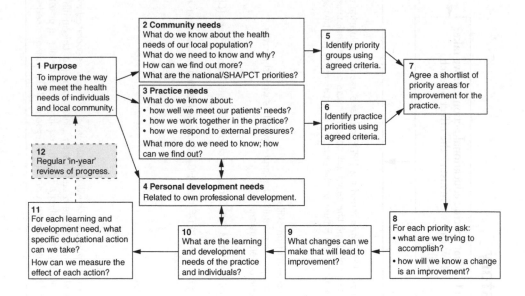

Planning for reviewing progress of the PPDP during the year

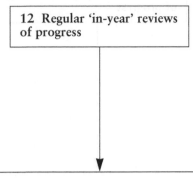

12 Regular 'in-year' reviews of progress

Regular review of progress is extremely important. Such reviews should achieve the following.

- Identify team members involved in the PPDP process and list those who are working together on specific areas of improvement (project groups).
- Identify those responsible for leading, co-ordinating and documenting the improvement and educational activities. Project groups should agree the frequency of their meetings and the frequency of feedback meetings to enable the PPDP project groups to present progress to the whole practice team. It is important to engage all members of the team in the PPDP. Wherever possible, try to fit reviews of progress into existing meetings.
- Allocate time for people to undertake the improvement priorities and to attend the appropriate educational opportunities.

You should be aware that this activity will change working and personal relationships.

The Maples Practice story

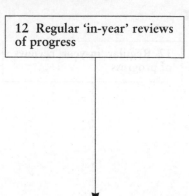

12 Regular 'in-year' reviews
of progress

The Maples Medical Centre PPDP team agreed the following schedule
of meetings in which to undertake their work, to feed back to the
PHCT, and to review the PPDP process:
- project groups would meet monthly initially (may become less
  frequent once the improvement work is underway)
- PPDP team would meet bi-monthly for one hour to review
  progress
- feedback would be provided to the whole PHCT at quarterly
  intervals.

Stage 6: Planning next year's PPDP

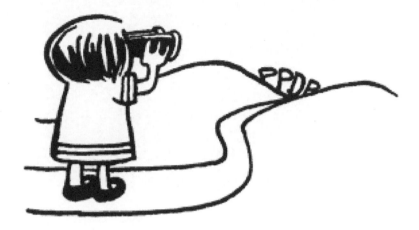

Purpose: To continue to improve the way that we meet the health needs of individuals, groups and the local community.

We suggest that a review be carried out nine to ten months into the plan (e.g. perhaps to coincide with the health authority or PCT planning timetable). Reviewing progress on your current plan will enable you to discuss and agree priorities for improvement for the next 12 months. You will also need to take into account the external agenda arising from national, SHA and PCT priorities including NSFs. For the purpose of reviewing the current plan it will be helpful to address the following questions for each priority area.

- With respect to the improvement priorities.
  - Did the planned improvement actions take place? If not, do you understand why?
  - If so what have been the outcomes? How do you know?
  - What has been learned from your PDSA feedback measures?
  - What have been the benefits – for patients and for staff?
- With respect to the educational actions.
  - Did the planned actions take place?
  - If so what have been the results? How do you know?
  - If the planned actions did not take place what were the barriers and difficulties? What has been learned from these and what further action has been, and needs to be, taken?
  - What have been the benefits – for patients and the staff involved?

Have any other internal or external priorities arisen, or been imposed, during the year which have led to revision of the plan? What are the implications of these for next year's PPDP?

Remember – this is a continuous process and the team will need to continually re-visit the framework, at least annually.

Stage 5: Planning next year's PDP

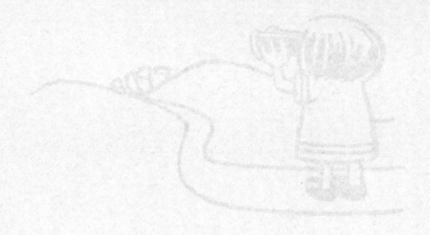

PART FOUR:

Some useful tips and resources

A guide to reflecting on the PPDP process

Checking out the team's understanding of the PPDP process is vital to enabling the group to progress confidently through the various stages. It is well worth taking 10 to 15 minutes at the end of each workshop to ask the group a few questions about their experience of the workshop and their developing understanding of PPDPs.

It is important to acknowledge that each practice will work at its own pace. Our experience has shown that with the assistance of an experienced facilitator much of the PPDP process can be completed in two two-and-a-half-hour workshops although this requires work to be undertaken between meetings as mentioned earlier. Some practice teams may choose to take longer and to spread the process over three or more workshops. The following are a few questions to help check out the team's understanding of the process.

At the end of each workshop check with participants how they felt the discussion had gone by asking:

• what went well
• what could have been better
• did you feel able to contribute to the discussion
• did you feel you were heard?

By the time you have completed Boxes 1, 2 and 3 of the PPDP process you may wish to discuss

- Participants' understanding of what a PPDP is.
- Participants' understanding of the purpose of the workshop.
- Whether there is a common understanding of the terms 'community needs' and 'practice needs' and whether the process to establish what these are has been effective.

By the time you have completed Boxes 5, 6 and 7 of the PPDP process you may wish to discuss

- Participants' understanding of the purpose of the workshop.
- Whether they feel that the chosen list of priorities reflects the needs of the practice's local population and its patients.

By the time you have completed Boxes 8, 9, 10 and 11 of the PPDP process you may wish to check

- Participants' understanding of the purpose of the workshop.
- Do they understand the framework for turning their priorities for improvement into action, i.e. the concept of CQI as described on pages 57–64?
- Do they understand the idea of testing series of small scale changes using the PDSA cycle, and its value?
- Are they clear how the identified team and individual learning needs link to the planned improvements?
- Are they clear about the links between PPDP and PDP?
- Was a timetable for regular review set up?

A brief introduction to the principles and methods of CQI*

CQI is a set of principles and methods that enables people to improve the processes and systems within which they work. At its core is the use of knowledge to identify changes, plan a test and assess the results. Its main driver is the desire to improve the match between the services professionals provide and the needs of the people who depend on them. These ideas are based on the premise that the foundation of quality is matching service to need and that quality improves as the match improves.[7] The principles and methods are currently the subject of much work within healthcare and learning from this work underpinned the team stories represented in this guide.[8]

Perhaps the first important message is that CQI is not a newly developed theory but is based on values and principles that are neither new nor controversial and with which most professionals are already familiar. What is perhaps new is the attempt to integrate them into a framework that can be used by practitioners in their everyday work to produce improvements that they themselves consider relevant to their clients/patients.

To improve care you need a model for providing care. At its simplest this is illustrated by the model in Figure 1.

Although simple the model has profound implications for service providers once it is unpicked. It makes connections between patient needs, outcomes measures that reflect these needs and the processes of care that link them. It is a universal model that applies equally well to health and community care, and begs many questions if we are to truly provide care that continuously improves the way it meets the needs of those who depend on it. In particular it raises questions about how we can understand and meet patient needs better, and how we can

* Adapted from Wilcock and Campion-Smith.[3]

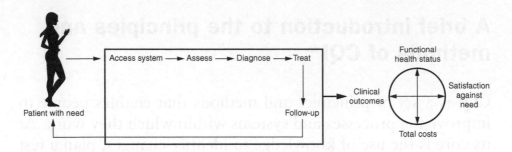

Figure 1: The model for providing care that underpins our work.[9]

develop outcome measures that reflect these needs. However this is beyond the scope of this guide. Our focus is on the use of CQI principles and methods to provide a very pragmatic approach to PPDP.

Improving processes of care

Much of the emphasis of published CQI studies to date has been on the middle part of the model, with professional teams working together to redesign the processes underpinning their practice.[10–12] This is critically important since it is impossible to improve care without improving the processes by which it is delivered. Teams discover, for example, that when they try to draw simple flowcharts describing the way they currently do things it stimulates much discussion about the assumptions on which they all operate. It is usually the first time that they have pooled their separate knowledge and used it to make joint decisions about where and how to improve the care they provide. This very patient-focused discussion seems to serve an important purpose in creating new ways of doing things that strengthens interprofessional teamworking.

However, there is also a need to look at each end of the care model.

Discovering patient needs

One currently emerging challenge is how to ensure that the processes being improved are relevant to the needs of their beneficiaries. Most contact with patients/clients has focused on measuring their satisfaction with the services they receive. However it is being acknowledged that this has had little impact on improving care per se. It has been hypothesised that this is because such measures tell us little about patients/clients or their needs.[13,14] More recent work is attempting to design methodologies which learn about patients' needs by listening to them tell stories about the impact of their illness on their lives, rather than answer questions about the services they received, listening to them as people rather than merely as patients.[15,16] By doing so service teams can identify for themselves the needs to which they can respond and can establish their own improvement priorities based on what they learn.

Building balanced sets of outcomes measures

The concept of the balanced set of measures as applied to organisations is not new.[17,18] More recently Nelson and colleagues have adapted the concept for clinical care describing what they refer to as the 'clinical value compass'.[9] The underlying principle is that because both health and healthcare are complex no single measure can provide a clear picture of critical areas of performance. Nelson *et al.* have pointed out that what is needed is a way to provide a fast comprehensive overview of a few critical measures. It is necessary to identify a set of measures relevant to a particular client/patient group which are considered to be significant by the staff group providing their care. One aspect of a balanced set of measures is to check that improvement in one area has not been at the expense of quality in another. The clinical value compass has its greatest impact when it is being used to drive improvement since it can translate into operational measures which can become the focus for team efforts.

The four elements of the clinical value compass are as follows.

- **Clinical outcomes** These may be considered to be direct consequences of interventions, e.g. signs, symptoms, complications etc.
- **Functional status** Measures of health status that provide insight into the impact of clinical outcomes on, for example, quality of life.
- **Satisfaction against need** The important factor here is the integration of need with the concept of satisfaction, thus making it patient-referenced as well as service-focused. Thus measures may relate to processes of care or the personal benefits realised by patients/clients and their families.
- **Costs** Where costs are recognised to be an outcome of care. They may be direct service costs or indirect social costs.

Building knowledge for improvement

Continuous improvement depends upon continuous learning and stories of successful improvement are inevitably stories of people learning together. This may be learning about the needs of their patients/clients, about the outcomes of the care they provide to these people or about the processes by which they provide this care. Reflecting on what they learn will provide clues to areas where improvements are necessary. Implementing changes and establishing key feedback measures creates another tier of learning and is at the heart of continuous improvement.

At this point it is worth noting what seem to be the two most important paradigms.

- Focusing on patient/client needs, which is close to the hearts of all professionals.
- Creating opportunities for adults to learn. Learning is a natural human ability and is fun despite any adverse experiences of education encountered during school and college careers.

When these two paradigms merge in practice settings, very powerful conditions for real and sustainable improvement exist. The PPDP guide is underpinned by these paradigms.

Having a framework for learning

Experience with improvement teams suggests that they benefit from having simple frameworks to guide them through their efforts. The framework that has received most attention recently is based on the work of Tom Nolan and his colleagues.[7] *See* Figure 2 for a diagrammatic representation.

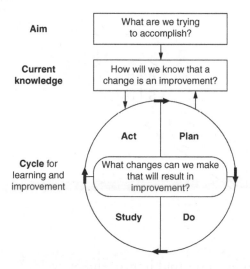

Figure 2: Model for improvement.[7]

The Nolan framework consists of three questions that offer a systematic way to turn ideas into action and increase the chances that it will lead to real improvements in practice. Addressing these questions leads to the PDSA cycle used as the guide to the implementation of, and learning from, the changes. As Berwick has noted, all improvement is change but not all change is improvement.[19] The Nolan questions are built into the PPDP framework and influenced the work of the different practice teams who tested it out. The PDSA cycle is congruent with the concept of action learning that underpins the PPDP process as described in Part Three of this guide.

As far as possible the idea is to choose small changes that can be implemented quickly. This is highly motivating for staff and the learning begins quickly thus maintaining their interest. Larger improvements are realised by the cumulative effects of rapid improvement (PDSA) cycles underpinned by serial learning (*see* Figure 3).[7]

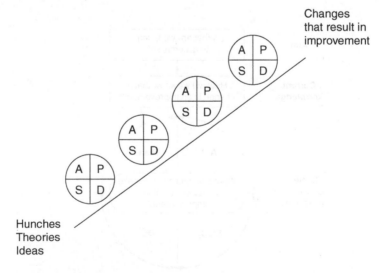

Changes that result in improvement

Hunches
Theories
Ideas

Figure 3: Serial learning and rapid improvement cycles.[7]

Broadly speaking the Nolan framework can be translated into the following major steps.[9]

1   Identify a specific group of patients/service users as the focus for enquiry.
2   Agree a high level, general aim.
3   Clarify what you currently know:
    • about these people and their needs
    • about the processes by which care is currently being provided (drawing a flowchart with your colleagues might be helpful)
    • from available data, e.g. audit results, complaints etc.
4   Use what you learn from the above to identify areas for improvement. Choose one or two to begin with.
5   Turn these improvement ideas into specific actions using the Nolan questions to begin PDSA cycles (*see* Figure 2). Make sure you build in simple feedback measures.
6   Use learning from the feedback to design further improvements using PDSA cycles as appropriate.

Some learning

We have learned much from our attempts to introduce CQI methods. Some key points are listed below.

• Topics must feel important. Ensuring they will produce benefits for patients/service users is important to initiating projects, whilst providing parallel benefits to staff is important to sustaining their interest and energy.
• Professionals from different professions learning together have great knowledge and understanding. No one person knows it all.
• Protected time is crucial. This produces initial reactions of horror but teams that have managed it consider it to have been worthwhile for patients/service users and to have benefits to working practice as well.

- Teams value structure and guidance to ensure that time spent is an investment.
- Improvement teams have fun.

Summary

Maintaining improvement teams is difficult due to very heavy workloads but progress will not be made unless protected time can be secured. It is critical therefore that time spent is an investment rather than a burden. This demands a clear focus on topics of importance to patients and the practice, and the use of frameworks that will guide activities to success. Combining the PPDP framework and process with the principles and methods of CQI described above seems to be very helpful in this respect. There is a crucial need for support and commitment to protected time from high levels within practices. In addition there is a need to ensure that this activity informs and complements PDPs. It would be well worthwhile considering how to offer academic recognition for time spent in PPDP activity so that learning improvement skills becomes a crucial part of professional education alongside the learning of professional and technical skills.[8]

For more detailed information about aspects of continuous quality improvement, see the NHS Modernisation Agency Improvement Leaders' Guides, www.modern.nhs.uk/improvementguides.

One practice's story of team learning with PPDP*

A market town practice (five principals, three whole time equivalents, 5700 patients) has been able to embrace the PPDP concept leading to significant patient benefits. The concept was launched at a multidisciplinary meeting. Ideas and information from this meeting were documented and circulated to all participants. The practice committed two hours of protected meeting time each month, replacing an unproductive previous meeting.

The process is led by the practice clinical governance lead who is a GP partner. Simple work sheets are produced for each team member and distributed seven days before meetings. These sheets advertise meeting time and location, advise on group work and have space for each person to log their notes from this working time. They are collated in PDPs and in a practice PPDP portfolio, providing an essential link between personal and group learning.

Meetings generally consist of work in small groups for the first hour, followed by lunch and feedback on work to the whole group. Significant event analysis or a short talk from a visiting speaker makes up the second part of the meeting.

The practice followed the PPDP framework described earlier in this guide. Their journey through the different stages is outlined below.

Agreeing the purpose (*see* Box 1 in the framework diagram)

There was agreement across the team that the purpose was to provide a high quality primary care service that meets patients'

---

* Much of this material was first published in the *British Journal of General Practice* and is used with permission of the editors.[20]

needs, both for care when they are unwell and to enable people to do all they can to remain healthy. Secondary aims of remaining a financially secure organisation and providing a good workplace for all staff were also agreed.

Assessing the needs (*see* Boxes 2, 3 and 4)

A number of needs were identified by staff at the initial meeting. Other imperatives have either arisen from audits or significant events ('internal'), or have come from government policy, health authority or PCT directives ('external'). It is also accepted that individuals within the team will have personal learning needs arising from questions in their own practice, reflection on their work or appraisal.

Negotiating the actions to take and sharing the work (*see* Boxes 5, 6 and 7)

The practice accepted that negotiation and choice was important – it would have been easy to take on too much and complete little. They looked for areas where there was congruence between the practice's aims and those things that 'had to be done' to satisfy the external agenda. They were also able to ensure the work was consistent with the practice's membership of the National Primary Care Collaborative.

Planning the actions (*see* Boxes 8 and 9)

For each action planned the practice team followed the CQI model and agreed:

• the high-level aim

- what specifically we are trying to accomplish
- the change that we think will lead to improvement
- the measurements to see if the change has resulted in improvement
- the plan to implement the change as a trial.

The practice team or sub group then entered the PDSA process.[9]

Identifying the learning needs (*see* Box 10)

For each change planned they looked to see what the learning needs were for the improvement to come about. These included:

- the acquisition of specific skills or knowledge by one or two team members, e.g. a practice nurse's learning about how to carry out spirometry and the interpretation of the results
- more general knowledge for a greater number of the team, e.g. all of the clinical team needed to know which patients it is appropriate to refer to spirometry, what the patient should expect and what the likely outcomes might be
- systems with which it was essential the whole team were confident, e.g. the use of a paperless internal communication and message system.

Planning learning actions (*see* Box 11)

Once these learning needs were identified, ways to meet them were decided upon. These included attendance at external courses, bringing a resource to a practice education meeting or just a learning activity within the team.

Some improvements planned, implemented and evaluated

- A protocol for the rapid management of simple urinary tract infection.
- The establishment of a palliative care register with fortnightly interprofessional meetings to review those patients on it.
- Establishing a spirometry service for patients with chronic lung disease.
- Changes to ensure practice prescribing costs remained within budget without loss of quality.
- A programme of regular resuscitation training for all staff.
- A practice team approach to increasing influenza vaccine uptake.
- A whole practice approach to meeting the NSF targets for coronary heart disease.
- The introduction of a 'Smokestop' clinic in the practice.
- Introduction of regular significant event analysis meetings to which any team member can propose a topic.
- Improved use of consistent coded computerised data for patient records and procedures to maintain the accuracy of these records.
- A number of initiatives to improve patient access including:
  - telephone surgeries
  - direct referrals of patients already assessed as needing specialist review by opticians
  - nurse consulting and triage plans for self measurement of blood pressure by selected patients
  - development of a practice website
  - a more flexible appointment system creating slots for 'semi-urgent' problems.

Specific examples of benefits from the PPDP

A fast track service for women with symptoms of simple urinary tract infection (UTI)

- **Aim** To use patient and staff time effectively to give safe and accessible care.
- **What are we trying to achieve?** To manage simple UTI safely, conveniently and effectively without a face-to-face consultation.
- **Can we plan a change that we think will lead to improvement?** A fast track service for patients with simple UTI that will allow them to receive appropriate treatment, provide a specimen and ensure accurate documentation.
- **Can we make measurements to see if the change has resulted in improvement?** Patient and staff satisfaction, review of notes to check documentation, review of drugs prescribed against subsequent bacteriology reports.
- **How can we plan to implement the change as a trial?** A small multidisciplinary working group devised a protocol. This was fed back to the whole team at a PPDP meeting and everyone agreed its value and limitations. The service was advertised and offered to patients. All patients with simple UTI symptoms were offered 'fast track' service for two months. Review of records of those using the service after two months and direct telephone enquiries were made of a sample to evaluate their levels of satisfaction.
- **What are the learning needs and actions required?** Review of evidence to allow writing of protocol, IT skills development to allow simple 'one keystroke macro' operation, training for reception staff in offering the service and administering the protocol questions.

Results

- **Benefits to patients**
  - improved access and treatment with minimum delay
  - released appointments
  - safe non-consultation prescribing ensured.
- **Benefits to team**
  - consistent recording in the medical record of the patient contact
  - widespread learning about the management of UTI
  - development of IT skills.

Establishing a palliative care register and regular review meetings

- **Aim** To work as an effective and supportive interprofessional clinical team.
- **What are we trying to achieve?** To improve patient care, interprofessional communication and teamworking and support in a practice-based team delivering palliative care.
- **Can we plan a change that we think will lead to improvement?** To establish a practice palliative care register and conduct a fortnightly interprofessional review of the patients on it.
- **Can we make measurements to see if the change has resulted in improvement?** Review after four months. Did the meetings occur? Are there instances where care improved as a result? Did staff members value the meetings?
- **How can we plan to implement the change as a trial?** Clinical team to meet regularly to review those on the register. Agreed criteria for entry to the register, agreed computer coding to record entry.
- **What are the learning needs and actions required?** Review of different criteria defining 'palliative care'. Dissemination to whole team of understanding of special needs of patients receiving palliative care and their families. Review of criteria for assessing care as a basis for regular review. Development of skills of membership and leadership of interprofessional team. Review of procedures used to ensure continuity of care out of hours. Specific clinical and communication issues identified for future learning as they arise.

Results

- **Benefits to patients**
  - review of their care and needs
  - team members more aware of their situation
  - criteria-based review of their care should lead to less unmet need
  - regular proactive review should lessen the chance of patients becoming 'lost'.
- **Benefits to team**
  - team members feel better supported in their work
  - there is a forum for discussing difficult clinical or interpersonal issues
  - there is an opportunity for specific learning in response to clinical problems.

Introducing nurse telephone consulting – learning actions

The whole practice team had been working together to improve access in line with the PCT and National Primary Care Collaborative targets. The team had considered a variety of ways in which to improve access including the introduction of some sort of triage system. For this to be effective it was decided that the introduction of nurse telephone consultations with patients requesting same day appointments or home visits would be appropriate.

A number of specific learning needs and actions were identified.

Two practice nurses with an interest in expanding their role were keen to join a locally-provided university course on nurse consulting. They also acknowledged that much of their learning would occur once they started to use the skills they had learned on the course and so protected time for routine review of all their telephone consultations by one of the partners was scheduled in.

The nurses were able to put this taught course and the subsequent reflection on this new aspect of their practice into their PDPs and portfolios.

The practice also recognised that nurse telephone consulting needed to be fully integrated into the work of the practice and the key role of the reception team in this. There was specific learning for the reception team on the role and benefits of nurse consulting and a chance to discuss and rehearse how the service would be offered to patients as an additional service rather than as a barrier to seeing the doctor.

The links between the PPDP and PDPs

Individual learning needs arising from the practice PPDP

The PPDP generated learning needs and actions. These were met in different ways:

- by the whole team working together
- by the team working individually on the same topic (e.g. everyone needing to update and maintain their resuscitation skills to the appropriate level)
- by individuals seeking specific training.

Personal learning arising from practice problems and its relationship to the PPDP

One GP's encounter with a patient who gave a history of Hepatitis C infection related to his previous intravenous drug use made the GP aware of how little he knew about the condition and its implications. The following excerpt from his PPDP illustrates the process of identifying the learning need and the subsequent actions.

Trigger event or area of uncertainty	Patient with history of Hepatitis C infection feeling unwell.
Learning need What do I need to find out/learn?	Learn more about Hepatitis C: clinical course, investigation, treatment, infectivity.
Learning plan How shall I do this? What will I do with whom, when?	Internet search, journal reading, ask colleagues.
The learning done What did I do?	• Web page of Canadian Association of Hepatology Nurses very useful, *Nursing Standard* review paper highlights high incidence of Hepatitis B and C carriers who are unaware of this. Suggests all patients should be treated as potentially infectious rather than depending on making value judgements – which may often be incorrect. • Discussion with local microbiology consultant has clarified significance and role of different tests – Liver Function Tests, core and surface antigen, polymerase chain reaction etc. • Discussion with recently-appointed consultant gastroenterologist who informs me that he has a special interest in the topic, is introducing a Hepatitis clinic locally with a nurse specialist and that he would be happy to review this patient but does not envisage any need for liver biopsy at present. • I learned more about clinical features including non-specific malaise, need for alcohol avoidance, risks of progressive disease and malignancy risk and role, and limitations of beta interferon and antiviral drugs.
Reflection What have I learned?	I now know the significance of the different tests (and have a written summary). I also have questioned my current policy and judgemental attitude to assessing infection risk. This has also highlighted the lack of practice-wide policy on wearing gloves for venepuncture.
Review Did I do the learning I planned? Did I find what I wanted? Has it altered my practice in any way? Is there any evidence of this for my portfolio? What next?	• I did the learning. • I found answers to the immediate question and now feel I know more about Hepatitis B and C. • I have reflected on the process and shared it with others as an example of informal 'just in time learning'. • I have questioned some of my judgemental decision making and have asked my partners to consider a practice-wide policy on routinely wearing gloves for venepuncture. • The written account of this learning journey is in my portfolio and has value for both process and content. • The initial patient has been referred to a specialist clinic.

Practicalities of drafting and implementing the PPDP: difficulties, barriers and solutions

Introducing a new task to an already beleaguered primary care team was not easy. The difficulty of finding a time when all the key people could meet, and the concern about the work building up while they were away from their usual work, was considerable. There was also a commonly held view that the PPDP meetings did not constitute 'real work' – only direct work with patients seems to fulfil this definition. There was a worry, arising from previous experiences, that the meeting would be a 'talking shop' and that nothing would be different for patients or staff as a result. There was some suspicion about the terminology or jargon used and concerns that the team was being expected to respond to someone else's agenda.

However the initial meetings were led in a way that ensured the staff felt a sense of ownership and control from the start. The initial issues chosen for action came from the internal agenda and some rapid improvement cycles with clear benefit for patients and staff helped overcome reservations. Once the staff had gained confidence in the process they felt happier to use it to respond to the external demands of the SHA and PCT priorities and NSFs.

Time remains a problem but it was emphasised that most of what the group dealt with was work that had to be done anyway and that the PPDP meetings provided an appropriate and efficient forum for getting the 'must do' tasks dealt with. Time was created by abandoning another regular meeting that had become protracted and of limited use. Nevertheless initial funding allowing payment of a locum to ensure the presence of key people has been important in establishing and sustaining the process. The lunchtime setting on a day when the reception team already meet and the provision of sandwiches has also helped.

However we believe the most important thing is that team members have felt involved in the selection of areas for improvement and in the planning and implementation of practical changes that they believe have improved the services for patients of the practice.

Key factors for success

- A process framework that made sense to all involved.
- Wholehearted willingness of the whole team (including attached and reception staff) to be involved and give it a try.
- A sense that this was helping do something they wanted to do anyway – meet their patients' needs better.
- Protected time initially to get the process going.
- An awareness of the need to manage the group process effectively.
- A practice member (the lead GP) who was willing to show great leadership and act as a champion for the initiative, both to start it off and maintain the momentum.
- Periodic review to make all aware of what has been achieved.

Enthusiasm for the process remains. The practice has decided not to run on a rigid annual cycle as different improvements and external imperatives to which it has to respond have differing timescales. Rather they view the PPDP process as a continually running mill of improvement that can be used to help the practice respond to a number of demands for change, be they externally imposed or arising from within.

The practice has linked the educational activities of individuals, small working groups and the whole team to meeting the needs of patients using a CQI approach.

They have found that their experience of shared learning to improve patient services is an effective use of time in a hard pressed practice team. Recognising the skills and potential of team members is consistent with current NHS policy. It also brings improvements in teamworking and relationships within the practice.

Personal development plans (PDPs)

We have said that PDPs are closely connected with PPDP and topics for personal learning and development may be identified as the team undertakes the PPDP process. However we have also acknowledged that individual team members may have interests, career plans and aspirations that will influence their learning plans. We believe the process of personal development planning can follow a similar framework to that which we propose for PPDPs.

As in PPDPs there needs to be a balance between responding to the external demands, reflection on personal practice and individual interests and aspirations. As with the PPDP, once an individual has identified the learning need, he or she will need to plan learning actions to meet that need with clear aims and measures to tell if each learning action has brought about the intended goal.

The framework given here is relevant for a variety of people working in the practice and is, we believe, as appropriate for a senior partner as for a practice nurse or GP registrar. By following the framework and gathering evidence of both the process followed and the learning achieved, we believe you will start an excellent foundation of materials on which to base Post Registration Education and Practice (PREP), appraisal and preparation for revalidation.

A framework of personal development planning

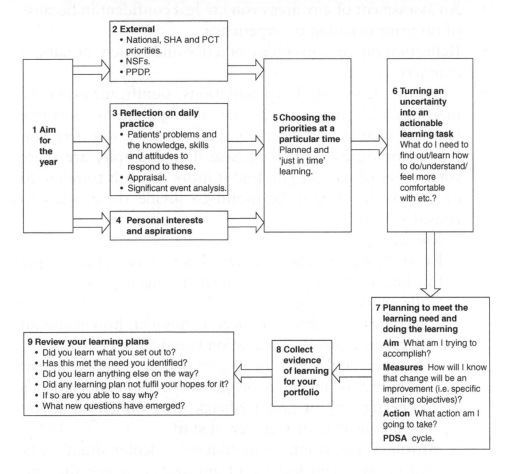

The following stages describe how you might build up the sections of your PDP portfolio as you follow this framework.

Stage 1: Discovering your needs (*see* Boxes 2–4)

You may wish to consider and include summaries of the following.

- National priorities, i.e. government directives such as 'Our Healthier Nation' and NSFs, and local documents, i.e. PCT Health Improvement Programme.

- Specific features of the practice and its population.
- An assessment of any areas you are less confident in because of no prior teaching or experience.
- Reflection on your everyday practice and review of patient contacts.
- Areas of uncertainty in consultations, significant events or meetings with an appraiser may all highlight areas where you feel unable to meet the patients' needs or where you feel uncomfortable or ill at ease. For example, are there some types of patient you find it more difficult to relate to or deal with? It may be useful to divide these areas to consider into:
  - **Knowledge**
  - **Know how**, i.e. who provides this service, where to get this information, how to contact this agency
  - **Skills** which may be:
    - **technical**, e.g. how to inject a shoulder, how to do an excision biopsy, resuscitation training
    - **interpersonal**, e.g. how to give bad news, make a visit after bereavement, challenge an unreasonable patient's expectations, or give feedback after unhelpful action by a colleague or member of staff
    - **Attitudes**, e.g. being aware that a particular situation or patient gives you feelings of annoyance, anger, discomfort, uncertainty or 'heartsink'.
- Results of audits or surveys of aspects of your practice such as timekeeping, casemix or prescribing.
- Issues that arise from regular appraisal and feedback from peers, partners or staff.

Use this section of your portfolio to log your learning needs.

Stage 2: Choosing areas for improvement and learning (*see* Box 5) (The 'what to do now' and 'why')

Planned learning

Some learning can be planned and may be best identified as a topic for personal study, a tutorial or a course.

Just-in-time learning

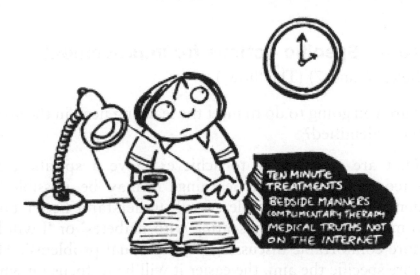

Much of our learning as adults is in response to real questions to which we need to know the answer. There is a lot of evidence that this sort of learning in response to a real need (and the discomfort of not knowing) can be very powerful and effective. This learning is often informal and quick – asking a colleague, using Mentor on the computer or *Clinical Evidence* or *BNF* on the desk or web. Sometimes we need to set aside a bit more time when we are aware that there is a larger gap in our knowledge.

Learning styles

You may be aware of your preferred and most effective learning style – there is wide variation. Be aware of the strengths and limitations of a single style and try to develop a range to suit different learning needs. You may decide that work on this is one of your early learning objectives. Questionnaires to help with this are available and your local GP Tutor will be able to guide you.

Use this section of your portfolio to record your choices for learning actions and why you made them.

Stage 3: Specific actions for improvement
(*see* Boxes 6 and 7) (The 'how')

What are you going to do to meet the learning need in the areas you have identified?

- What are you hoping to achieve? Have a specific aim/ outcome for successful learning. It may be possible to identify this, for example, 'I will understand better how to manage a patient presenting with diabetes' or 'I will be more comfortable discussing psychosexual problems'. The more specific the aim, the easier it will be to focus on what you need to do to achieve it.
- Identify measures that will tell you if you have achieved the goal – it could be a mini audit or a case review of one or more patients. How will you know that any changes you make are an improvement?
- Use the PDSA cycle to help you plan the changes, take the necessary action, evaluate the outcome and act upon the results.

Use this section of your portfolio to set out a plan of action: what learning; when you will do it; who or what will be the resources for this; when you will review the learning plan and with whom?

Stage 4: Building your portfolio (*see* Box 8)

Any evidence of what you have learned and any medium can go in your portfolio, including the following examples.

*   Patient case reviews.
*   Certificates from, and written reflections on, courses.
*   Summaries of articles read and how they will alter your daily practice.
*   Accounts of learning from personal contact and in small groups.
*   Practice policies written or papers presented to the practice at team meetings.
*   Reflections on discussion with colleagues.
*   If consultation skills are included as a learning area you might even want to include an audio or video tape of the consultation, but be aware of the rules relating to patient consent, safe storage and subsequent deletion of such confidential material.

Stage 5: Reviewing your learning plans
(*see* Box 9)

The commitment to review your plan is really important. The timescales of different learning activities will vary but you need to put time aside to make the review both by yourself and with someone else throughout the year. Even where you have not achieved what you set out to do, you will have learned something important – even if it is only about the things that can get in the way. Often at the review new learning objectives will be identified, but don't forget to acknowledge all you have achieved.

An excerpt from a personal portfolio might look like this:

Trigger event or area of uncertainty	Beta blockers in heart failure (HF). Patient discharged on beta blocker. I thought they were contraindicated in HF but have seen a paper somewhere on this.
Learning need What do I need to find out/learn?	Lots, on: • what is the evidence? • who benefits? • which drugs and what dose?
Learning plan How shall I do this? What will I do with whom when?	Internet journal search, look out for clinical meetings, ask colleagues.
Date and time spent learning	One hour Internet search and two hours' journal reading: 22.2.01.
Reflection What have I learned?	I now know the NYHA classification of HF. I know beta blockers are effective in selected patients with HF with benefit increasing over three months.
Review Did I do the learning I planned? Did I find what I wanted?	Yes, but need to do more.
Has it altered my practice in any way?	Have started one patient Mr PK – no clear benefit yet. May need to do an audit to think how many more should be considered. Add NYHA code to computer.
Is there any evidence of this for my portfolio? What next?	Discuss with practice team.

Simple log sheet for recording areas of uncertainty to prompt future learning

Problem or uncertainty	What do I need to know?	How will I find out?	Did I? (Date and person)	What have I learned?

Facilitating PPDP meetings: learning from our experience

The PPDP process enables:

- team members to learn both individually and as a team through a formally structured event and more informally through the daily course of their work
- practices to develop a positive attitude towards learning and to experience the value of learning together in an informal setting
- the team to create a learning culture and to plan strategically for the learning needs of individuals and for the needs of the team as a whole.

Facilitating your own practice team can be difficult – as a member of the team you have a contribution to make; as a facilitator you do not. To perform the role of facilitator and participant is to 'break the rules'; facilitators should remain totally impartial.[21] Practices may consider a reciprocal arrangement with a neighbouring practice based on trust and impartiality. Our experience has been that team learning is enhanced when the facilitator comes from outside the organisation and is able to focus entirely on the teams' needs, raising the feeling of safety in the group and allowing for more disclosure and risk taking.[22]

Practice teams are well known for status hierarchies – GP and employer can be perceived as dominant and powerful, nurses may be perceived as subservient and administrative staff can often be ignored. Each team member's contribution to the workshops will be determined by their job role and previous experiences. This requires the facilitator to be flexible in their approach and to be able to work with the emerging material – in other words to go with the flow.

Management of group dynamics is dependent on the skills of the facilitator who has the responsibility to create a comfortable and safe environment where all contributions are equally valued.

Initial meeting between facilitator and practice

The facilitator meets with the practice manager and sometimes one of the GPs to:

- discuss the PPDP process and agree dates and venues for the workshops
- ensure 'dedicated time out' to avoid people coming in late or leaving early
- encourage the practice to invite at least one representative from each discipline to attend (practice teams have varied in size from six to 26).

Preparation for the first meeting

It is important that people come to the first meeting with a clear idea of what it is about and we suggest some preparatory work to help them focus on the purpose of the meeting.

- It helps if each person attending is given a copy of the PPDP framework, together with a brief explanation of what the team is trying to achieve at the workshops.
- Check out everyone's understanding of 'community needs' – you may need to explain this beforehand.
- To establish 'practice needs' you could ask each member of the practice team to express an opinion on the current performance of the practice by using the SWOT (*see* pp 88–90) exercise or other similar tool. The results can be summarised and shared at the first meeting. There may be issues arising from the SWOT which may be important,

but not necessarily significant – these should be noted and addressed separately.

The first workshop

When the team comes together for the first workshop it is important to spend some time establishing an environment in which people can share views openly.[23,24]

- It is useful to ask the team to state their hopes, expectations and concerns about the whole process and record these on a flipchart. They will be surprised by how many feelings they share.
- The team can then work together to draw up some group agreements or ground rules about how they want the meeting to be conducted. It is vital that the group creates its *own* rules. Doing this exercise together is the first step to working/learning together. However, it is useful for the facilitator to have a checklist in case important items are forgotten, such as timekeeping, breaks and finish times.
- Congratulate the team on their first shared learning experience.

Starting the process

Begin by briefly explaining the PPDP framework diagram; it is always useful to reinforce the message and check out understanding. The team is then ready to work through the process.

- Check out the team's perception of 'community needs'. What are the issues for this practice? Note these on a flipchart.
- Present the outcome of the co-ordinated SWOT analysis and allow discussion, again making notes on the flipchart.
- Ask the team to split into small, mixed professional groups (of no more than four to five; if the practice is a small team this can be done as one group).
- Based on what they have heard/learned so far, ask the small groups to agree a list of priority areas for improvement.
- Bring the groups back together and ask them to present their lists. Note these on the flipchart.
- Working with the whole team, and with their agreement, narrow the list to a manageable number – usually two to three priority areas for improvement.
- Ask for volunteers to form small project groups to work on producing action plans (PDSA cycles) for each of the areas for improvement. Ensure these are mixed professional groups. Don't forget to ask the team to include people who may not be present at the workshop.
- Agree a date for the team to reconvene (usually four to six weeks later) to share their action plans and to work through the second part of the framework.

The second workshop

Begin by 're-forming' the group.
- Check for newcomers and absentees.
- Reconfirm the team's agreed ground rules.

- Agree a finish time.
- Ask the project groups to present their action plans and allow discussion from the team.
- Ensure the action plans follow the PDSA cycle and in particular include ways of measuring that the actions, once taken, have brought about improvement.
- Ask the team to split into small, mixed professional groups to discuss and agree what learning needs to take place in order to bring about the improvement and how this learning can be achieved.
- Remind the groups at this stage that they should also consider what may be appropriate for inclusion in individual learning plans.
- Bring the small groups back together and ask them to share their findings.
- Reach agreement on the learning plan for the practice and for individuals.
- Ask the group to consider how they plan to disseminate the PPDP to other members of the PHCT and to produce a timetable for regular review of progress.
- Set a date for annual review and planning of next year's PPDP.

SWOT analysis

SWOT is a tool for scrutinising an organisation and its environment.[25,26] It is the first step to helping teams focus on key issues. Once key issues have been identified they feed into the organisation's plan.

SWOT stands for strengths, weaknesses, opportunities and threats. Strengths and weaknesses are internal factors. For example, a strength could be your new purpose-built surgery. A weakness could be high staff turnover. Opportunities and threats are external factors. For example, an opportunity could be a new housing estate in your catchment area. A threat could be increased workload.

A word of caution – SWOT analysis can be very subjective. If you are presenting a summary of SWOT analyses as a foundation for your first workshop take care to present these as common issues, which have been identified by several members of the team.

The purpose of the SWOT exercise is to seek the views of each member of the PHCT on their perceptions of the practice. This can be undertaken as a practice team, as individuals or in unidisciplinary groups. The important issue is to ensure that everyone's views are sought.

Below are a few questions to guide you through the SWOT process.

Strengths

- What do we do well? (You will get an indication from patient surveys, prescribing data, performance indicators, audits, significant events.)
- How well do we work together as a team (not just get along)?
- Do we have special skills and expertise?
- Acknowledge the good things in your practice.

Weaknesses

- What don't we do well? (Use the indicators above to identify areas for improvement.)
- How good is teamworking and communication?
- Do we lack certain skills or expertise?
- Recognise the not-so-good things in your practice.

Opportunities

- Do we have an opportunity to change things?
- What can we do to meet national and local priorities?
- What opportunity do we have to improve our care for patients and our team?

Threats

- What gets in the way?

For further information about SWOT analysis there are a number of useful websites. For example try www.buzgate.com/vt_bft _swot.html.

Significant event analysis (SEA): a summary*

SEA is defined as occurring when:

> ... individual episodes in which there has been a **significant** occurrence (either beneficial or deleterious) are analysed in a **systematic** and detailed way to ascertain what can be learnt about the overall **quality of care** and to indicate changes that might lead to future **improvements**.

(after Pringle)[28]

It is an interprofessional team activity. There will be regular meetings to discuss events (both good and not-so-good). The focus is on system improvement rather than individual improvement. The development of a 'no blame' culture is essential.

SEA is part of the culture of clinical governance, risk management and the determination of learning needs. It promotes a positive approach to complaints, identifies audit and research topics, helps develop understanding of others' roles, and builds and develops the skills of teams.

Outcomes of SEA

There are five principal outcomes.

- **Congratulation.**
- **Immediate action** It is clear during the discussion at the meeting what needs to be done.
- **Conventional audit** To answer 'how often is this happening?'.

---

* We are grateful to Drs Richard Westcott, Grace Sweeney and Jonathan Stead, colleagues at Exeter University, for sharing their experience with introducing significant event analysis to primary care teams. Much of what follows is based on their work.[27]

- **Small group task** Discussion identifies a piece of work which needs to be done by two or three members of the team. The work will take place before the next meeting, but tackling the task during the SEA meeting would not be a good use of the team's time. The task may be a quality improvement project, production (or adaptation) of guidelines etc.

- **No action – 'Life is like that'** It is sometimes necessary to accept that such an event will sometimes happen and there is not much we can do about it.

Please don't forget the congratulations

There is not enough of it about. There is little history of praise in the NHS – just individual blame. There is usually some part of even an adverse event that is well managed and should be acknowledged.

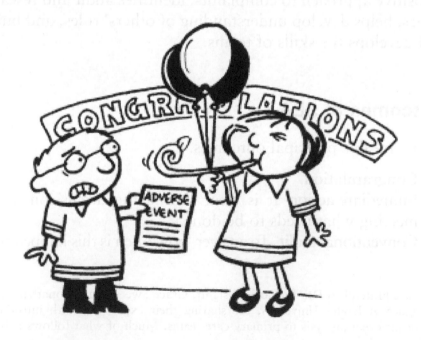

Managing the process

Management of the SEA process with good facilitation and leadership is essential. There must be commitment and ownership by the whole team, whose initial reservations should be expressed and heard. Reassurance, engendering a feeling of safety and assuring all that everyone will be able to participate in decision making is important. Agreement of rules and guidelines for the meetings may be important for this. The aim is to create small but important changes.

When the process works well it helps the team reach solutions and actions, and engenders a feeling of working together.

Topics should usually be presented by those involved with the significant event. Facilitated team discussion should start with praise for what went well before any criticism follows. Key points and actions should be recorded for future review.

The sensitive selection of topics, with some censoring and vetting of those not best dealt with in an open forum, is essential.

Examples of significant events

- Successful management of a crisis.
- Sudden unexpected death of a practice patient.
- Under-age pregnancy.
- Violence to staff.
- Drug errors and drug reactions.
- Complaints.
- Breaches of confidentiality.
- Buildings problems, security or health and safety issues.

Benefits of SEA

- Leads to change rapidly.
- Built into the fabric of the organisation.
- Systematic approach.
- Encourages a user/patient focus.
- Includes successes as well as problems.
- Fits well with the discovery of learning needs for a PPDP and individual PDPs.

Getting started

At least one member of the team should have skills and training in the facilitation of small group work.

- Initial meeting: invite and involve all stakeholders.
- Identify the chairman/manager.
- Meet monthly – instead of existing meetings, not as well.
- Collect events as they occur. Ensure all in the team know they can nominate events.
- Record events using forms or books kept in strategic places.
- If an event is described in a letter from another organisation, record the details.

Before the meeting

- Collect events a week prior to the meeting.
- Create agenda, recognising:
  - priority of topics
  - availability of personnel
  - involvement of team members
  - sensitivity of topic
  - flexibility to add 'hot topics'.
- Circulate agenda 48 hours before meeting.

At the meeting

- Run through the minutes of the last meeting, in particular the action points.
- Each topic should be presented by the key person, followed by discussion (praise before criticism).
- Ensure the discussion does not dominate the meeting and make the agenda unachievable.
- Check the course of action is approved by the team.
- Record the key points and actions decided, and by whom.

Maintaining and sustaining the process

- A healthy and varied agenda.
- Monitor the overall process on a six-monthly basis. Review the topics covered and the outcomes.
- Look at the changes achieved. Have they improved things for staff or patients?
- Ask how people *feel* about the process and their participation.
- Review the timing of meetings. Is anyone excluded?
- Summarise actions at the end of the meeting.
- Increase the number of congratulations.
- Don't forget the congratulations.

Further information can be found on the website http://latis.ex.ac.uk/sigevent/.

References

1 Wilcock PM, Campion-Smith C and Head M (2002) The Dorset Seedcorn Project: interprofessional learning and continuous quality improvement in primary care. *Br J Gen Pract.* **52**: S39–44.

2 Department of Health (1998) *A Review of Continuing Professional Development in General Practice: a report by the Chief Medical Officer.* DoH, London.

3 Wilcock PM and Campion-Smith C (2002) Using the principles and methods of continuous quality improvement within the RIPE project. In: L Todres and K Macdonald (eds) *Making it Better: improving health and social care through interprofessional learning and practice development.* Bournemouth University, Bournemouth.

4 Campion-Smith C, Smith H, White P *et al.* (1998) Learners' experience of continuing medical education events: a qualitative study of GP principals in Dorset. *Br J Gen Pract.* **48**: 1590–3.

5 Department of Health (2000) *A Health Service of All the Talents: developing the NHS workforce: consultation document on the review of workforce planning.* DoH, London.

6 Wilcock P and Headrick L (2000) Interprofessional learning for improvement of health care: why bother? *J Interprofessional Care.* **14**: 2.

7 Langley GJ, Nolan KM, Nolan TW *et al.* (1996) *The Improvement Guide.* Jossey Bass Publishers, San Francisco, CA.

8 Batalden PB and Stoltz PK (1993) A framework for the continual improvement of healthcare: building and applying professional and improvement knowledge to test changes in daily work. *Joint Commission J Quality Improvement.* **October**: 424–52.

9 Nelson EC, Batalden PB and Ryer J (eds) (1998) *Clinical Improvement Action Guide.* Joint Commission on Accreditation of Healthcare Organisations, Chicago, IL.

10   Cox S, Wilcock P and Young J (1999) Improving the repeat prescribing process in a busy general practice: a study using continuous quality improvement methodology. *Quality in Health Care.* 8: 119–25.

11   Headrick L, Katcher W, Neuhauser D *et al.* (1994) Continuous quality improvement and knowledge applied to asthma care. *Joint Commission J Quality Improvement.* 20(10): 562–8.

12   Neuhauser D, McEachern JE and Headrick L (1995) *Clinical CQI: a book of readings.* Joint Commission on Accreditation of Healthcare Organisations, Chicago, IL.

13   Gustafson DH, Taylor JO, Thompson SP *et al.* (1993) Assessing the needs of breast cancer patients and their families. *Quality Management in Health Care.* 2(i): 6–17.

14   Guaspari J (1998) The hidden costs of customer satisfaction. *Quality Digest.* **February:** 45–7.

15   Department of Health (2001) *Coronary Heart Disease Collaborative Toolkit: learning from patient and carer experiences.* NHS Modernisation Agency, London.

16   McKinley ED (2000) Under toad days: surviving the uncertainty of cancer recurrence. *Ann Internal Med.* **133**(6): 479–80.

17   Kaplan RS and Norton DP (1992) The balanced scorecard: measures that drive performance. *Harvard Business Rev.* **January–February:** 71–9.

18   Kaplan RS and Norton DP (1993) Putting the balanced scorecard to work. *Harvard Business Rev.* **September–October:** 134–42.

19   Berwick DM (1996) A primer on leading the improvement of systems. *BMJ.* **312:** 619–22.

20   Campion-Smith C and Riddoch A (2002) One Dorset practice's experience of using a quality improvement approach to practice professional development planning. *Br J Gen Pract.* **52:** S33–7.

21   Boud D, Keogh R and Walker D (eds) (1985) *Reflection: turning experience into action.* Kogan Page, London.

22   Elston S (2002) *Educational Facilitator Project Report.* Institute of Health and Community Studies, Bournemouth University.

23 Jones RVH (1992) Getting better: education and the primary healthcare team. *BMJ*. **305**: 506–8.

24 Spiegal N, Murphy E, Kinmonth AL *et al.* (1992) Managing change in general practice: a step by step guide. *BMJ*. **304**: 231–4.

25 Bartol KM and Martin DC (1991) *Management*. McGraw Hill, New York.

26 Johnson G, Scholes K and Sexty RW (1989) *Exploring Strategic Management*. Prentice Hall, Scarborough, Ontario.

27 Westcott R, Sweeney G and Stead J (2000) Significant event audit in practice: a preliminary study. *Family Practice*. **17**(2): 173–9.

28 Pringle M, Bradley CP, Carmichael CMA *et al.* (1995) Significant event auditing: a study of the feasibility and potential of case-based auditing in primary medical care. *Occasional Paper, Royal College of General Practitioners*. **70**: i–viii, 1–71.

Index

actions
  agreeing specific 42–5
  improvement 42–5
  planning 66–7
approach 21–3

background 20–1
barriers 74–5
benefits
  PPDPs 69–71
  SEA 94

Calman, Sir Kenneth 9, 20
clinical outcomes, clinical value
    compass component
    59–60
clinical value compass
    59–60
community needs 28, 36–8, 39,
    42, 47–9, 50
congratulations 91, 92
contents, this guide 15–16
context 20–1
continuous quality improvement
    (CQI) 29
  key points 63–4
  methods 57–76
  model 57–8
  principles 57–76
costs, clinical value compass
    component 59–60
CQI *see* continuous quality
    improvement
cycle, PPDP 34

decision-making processes, linking
    21–3
development needs, agreeing
    46–9
difficulties 74–5
discovering patient needs 59
drafting PPDPs 74–5

education, modernising 20–1
evaluation, improvement 68
evidence, portfolio, PPDP 38, 41,
    44–5, 49
examples
  benefits, PPDPs 69–71
  SEA 92
  team learning 65–8

feedback 10, 14, 23–4
framework
  learning 61–3
  PDPs 77–83
  PPDPs 27–34
function, this guide 19–26
functional status, clinical value
    compass component
    59–60

implementation
  improvement 68
  PPDPs 74–5
improvement
  achieving 46–9
  actions 42–5, 80
  care processes 58–9

choosing areas for 39–41,
      79–80
evaluation 68
implementation 68
model for 61–3
planned improvement projects
      28, 29, 68
interprofessional meetings 30–1

key success factors 75
knowledge building 60–1

learning
   choosing areas for 79–80
   just-in-time 79
   planned 79
   styles 80
learning needs
   agreeing 46–9
   identifying 29, 67
   individual 29, 71–3
   linking 46–9
   PPDPs and PDPs 71–3
   practice team 29
learning process 18
learning, team 65–8
linking, decision-making processes
      21–3
links, PPDPs and PDPs 71–3

Maples Practice
   actions for improvement 44–5
   areas for improvement 41
   development needs 47–9
   learning needs 47–9
   priority needs 38
   progress review 52
meetings
   facilitating 84–8
   initial 84, 94–5
   interprofessional 30–1

preparation 85–6
   review 33–4, 70
models
   CQI 57–8
   for improvement 61–3

needs
   agreeing 66
   discovering patients' 59
   discovering priority needs 36–8
   PDPs 77–8
   see also community needs;
      learning needs; personal
      development needs; practice
      needs
negotiation 66
Nolan framework 61–3

objectives, this guide 16, 23–4
opportunities, SWOT analyses 90
outcomes
   clinical 59–60
   SEA 91–2
outcomes measures, balanced sets
      59–60

palliative care register 70
participants' understanding
      55–6
patient needs, discovering 59
PCTs see primary care trusts
PDPs see personal development plans
PDSA see plan-do-study-act
personal development needs 28,
      36–8, 39, 42, 47–9, 50
personal development plans
      (PDPs) 76–83
   framework 77–83
   and PPDPs 25–6
PHCT see primary healthcare
      team

plan-do-study-act (PDSA) 43–5, 61–3
planned improvement projects 28, 29, 68
planning
  actions 66–7
  and development 20–1
  learning 79, 81–3
  PPDPs 53
portfolio, PPDP 31–4
  building 81, 82
  evidence 38, 41, 44–5, 49
PPDPs *see* Practice Professional Development Plans
practicalities 74–5
practice needs 28, 36–8, 39, 42, 47–9, 50
Practice Professional Development Plans (PPDPs), defined 19
preparation 18
primary care trusts (PCTs), linking 23
primary healthcare team (PHCT) 23–4
priorities
  discovering needs 36–8
  groups 40–1
  identifying 28–9, 32, 40–1
  practice 40–1
  shortlist 40–1
  translating 28, 29
process
  maintaining 95
  managing 93
  starting 87, 94
  sustaining 95
professions, characteristics 7
progress, review 33–4, 50–2

purpose 28, 36–8, 39, 42, 47–9, 50
  agreeing 65–6
  this guide 19–26

recommendations 20–1
references 97–9
reflecting, on PPDP process 55–6
requirements 20–1
resources 41–95
review
  learning plans 81–3
  meetings 33–4, 70
  progress 33–4, 50–2

satisfaction against need, clinical value compass component 59–60
SEA *see* significant event analysis
self regulation 7
significant event analysis (SEA) 91–2
  benefits 94
  examples 93
solutions 74–5
stages, PPDP process 28, 31–2, 35–53
strengths, SWOT analyses 89
SWOT analyses 32, 40–1, 85, 88–90

team learning, examples 65–8
team working 20–1
telephone consulting 71
threats, SWOT analyses 90
time, constraint 8, 23–4, 74–5
tips 41–95
training, modernising 20–1

underlying thoughts 19–26
understanding, participants'
        55–6
urinary tract infection (UTI), fast
        track service 69
using this guide 17
UTI *see* urinary tract infection

weaknesses, SWOT analyses 89
work-sharing 66
workforce, planning and
        development 20–1
workshops
    first 86
    second 87–8

T - #0682 - 101024 - C0 - 246/174/6 - PB - 9781857758054 - Gloss Lamination